WOMEN
—*Who Do*—
Too Much

Stress and the Myth of the Superwoman

Patricia H. Sprinkle

HarperPaperbacks
New York, New York
ZondervanPublishingHouse
Grand Rapids, Michigan
Divisions of HarperCollinsPublishers

HarperPaperbacks   *A Division of* HarperCollins*Publishers*
                    10 East 53rd Street, New York, N.Y. 10022

A trade paperback edition of this book was published in
1992 by ZondervanPublishingHouse, a division of
HarperCollins*Publishers*.

First HarperPaperbacks printing: February 1996

Printed in the United States of America

HarperPaperbacks, ZondervanPublishingHouse, and
colophon are trademarks of HarperCollins*Publishers*

❖ 10 9 8 7 6 5 4 3 2 1

WORDS OF A
Wise Woman

"God doesn't want you busy
about everything.
God does want you busy
about something.
God even knows what it is."
(p. 22)

"If you don't decide how to
spend your life,
somebody else will decide for you."
(p.59)

"If you don't know where you
want to go,
you'll never know whether you
get there."
(p.78)

"Besides the noble art of
getting things done,
there is the noble art of leaving
things undone."
(p.86)

To Bob,
who sometimes eases my stress
and sometimes adds to it,
but always lives up to his
marriage vow to enable my
life's mission as his own.

Contents

WOMEN
—*Who Do*—
Too Much

Preface

This book is written to all women who are doing too much and know it. It is written to end the myth that just because something needs doing, you personally have to do it. It is written to help you begin to discover, with God's help, precisely what *you* have been created to be and do—and how to limit yourself to being and doing only that. As you read this book and work through the exercises after each chapter, I pray that you will begin to live not more efficiently, but more effectively.

The book was born when I was asked to lead a workshop on "Stress and the Christian Superwoman." At that time I was working full time for the Presbyterian Hunger Program out of my Georgia home, commuting one week a month to our Kentucky headquarters, traveling frequently to hunger meetings around the nation, completing my second mystery novel, mothering two boys (eight and eleven), and giving some assistance to my husband as he pastored a local congregation. I was not, however, particularly stressed, and there was no invisible superwoman cape in my closet.

Fifteen years before, I was swamped by stress. Convinced that I had to perform any good task and work on any good issue that came my way, I was constantly overwhelmed by guilt, because no matter how much I did, I never could do enough. At last I cried out to God for relief. God put me in a school of the Spirit designed to take a look at time and what it is really for. In the years since, I have discovered principles and processes that enable me to limit what I do, and to do it at a manageable, often leisurely, pace.

I felt, therefore, I had something to teach—not answers or a surefire formula, but principles and processes that can help other women, with God's help, manage their own lives and reduce their stress. These principles and processes apply to women in homes, offices, and churches. They apply to women who are single or married, women with children or without, women who are young or old. The principles may apply even to men. I chose to write to women because I know their stresses firsthand.

After the workshop, several women asked me to put these principles and processes in writing. Again asking God's help, I agreed to try. God responded to my request with divine humor.

In the time that I was writing this book, God's "help" did not result in flowing prose and completed chapters. Instead, God let our family's stress increase. Bob lost his job. My interim job ended. Our basement flooded to the doorknobs. After almost a year of unemployment, Bob found a new job in Florida. He moved in April, leaving me a single parent until school was out. We moved the weekend of my college reunion, so he drove the truck to Florida while I flew to New York. We left a home we had designed and built, and we moved into one with a single upstairs air conditioner; I wrote through a Florida summer with my door open to lonely children in a new town. Two bikes were stolen. Six weeks after I got to Florida, Bob was called to serve a church in Alabama. He moved in September and I remained behind to complete this book, once again juggling children's needs with appointments with realtors. Each night I wondered: What will tomorrow bring?

Don't feel sorry for me, however. That's how life is sometimes. Those eighteen months demonstrated that the principles I discuss in these chapters really work. I was busy, even harried. I wasn't overwhelmed.

When I joked that God was increasing my stress to test my principles, my very wise thirteen-year-old said, "No, Mama, God is saying, "You think *you* got stress? I've got the whole universe to run, full of drug dealers, hungry people, war, and earthquakes. You want to talk about stress—I'll show you stress!' No matter how bad it gets for us, Mama, it's always worse for God."

Thanks, Barnabas, I needed that. We all need to remember that no matter how bad our own stress gets, other people (and God) have more. Between them, God and my children have made this a very honest book.

God also provided a special gift. Within one two-week period, I had the opportunity to interview fourteen other women, some new friends and some whom I have long admired for the amount they accomplish with so little visible stress. What they had to say has greatly enriched this book. You will learn about them as you meet them in the pages of these chapters as well as through the short biographical sketches I have included in Appendix B.

Find a quiet place and take your Bible, a pencil, and a legal pad or notebook (you'll need that much paper). Spend a whole day or several quiet mornings reading and praying through these pages. God has some surprises in store for you. You don't have to do it all!

CHAPTER ONE

All Things to All People

Are you always busy yet never feel you get enough done?

Do you set goals for yourself then get so swamped meeting other people's needs that you fail to accomplish those goals?

Do you make resolutions—"I'll lose ten pounds," "I'll spring clean my house," "I'll get a more fulfilling job"—and find the primary result is one more layer of guilt?

If so, you are a perfectly normal stressed-out woman.

These days women still do most of the cooking, cleaning, laundry, and volunteer work. We bear the children and in most cases have primary responsibility for raising them. Mothers chauffeur and bake for school parties. Wives act as partner and social hostess for husbands. Over half of all married women now have part-time or full-time jobs as well. Single mothers cope alone with finances, family schedules, crises, homemaking, and full-time work. Childless, single, and widowed women are pressured to give longer hours to work or to charitable organizations because "you don't have a family to care for"—then are subtly (often not-so-subtly!) pressured to get one.

For Christian women the problem can be even more acute. We add church activities—teaching Sunday school, chairing committees, leading Bible study groups, serving soup at shelters, and singing in the choir—to already busy schedules. We try to be "cheerful givers" who joyfully present our bodies as living sacrifices. But our bodies are so tired! Whatever happened to the love, joy, peace, and those other fruits of the Spirit promised in Galatians 5:22—23? For many Christian women today, the only fruit of the Spirit they experience is long-suffering!

Because most of us have, to one extent or another, believed the myth that we are *supposed* to be super-women, our weariness is intensified by guilt. A study of six women attending a college reunion revealed only one thing in common after twenty years: while some were married and some were not, some had children and others did not, some worked at home and some had outside careers, they were uniformly stressed by guilt. Why? Because not one of them felt that she was doing enough. Does that sound familiar?

How many of us rise each morning and don our superwoman capes, spend our days trying to do everything anybody expects us to do (and a few things we want to do, as well), and fall into bed at night counting the things we failed to get done and convinced that our stressed-out feeling is a shameful, personal weakness?

Actually, we are stressed out for a very good reason: God never intended us to be superwoman. Nor were we designed to live by stress alone.

Stress itself is God-given. We are designed so that when we meet a situation that requires more energy than we normally have, our bodies produce extra hormones and blood sugars to make us equal to the task. That's how we get through the last hours of a grueling meeting, the last pushes of childbirth, and the pots and pans after Thanksgiving dinner. But when the surge of hormones and additional sugar recedes, we are left feeling drained—even if we enjoyed what we were doing. That is why we feel as exhausted after bringing home a new baby, getting a longed-for promotion, or spending a day at the beach as we do after a harried day at work or a week with the chicken pox.

When stress operates as it is supposed to, we face challenges, have energy to meet them, then collapse with our feet up before going on to something else. What wears us out—and what most of the time we identify as "stress"—is day after day of too many challenges to meet and too much to do.

One women's group was discussing how overwhelmed we all were by life's demands. We had just concluded that we didn't really believe God intended us to live such hectic, chaotic lives, when one woman asked in all innocence, "But doesn't the Bible say that we are to be all things to all men?" (That verse, we decided, is one good argument for inclusive language in Bible translations.)

We also agreed that this is only one of many verses

3

that Christian women use to explain why we stay so busy. We think we are *supposed* to be "all things to all people."

A closer look at 1 Corinthians 9:22, however, reveals that how we live our lives is the opposite of what Paul did. He writes, "I have become all things to all men so that by all possible means I might save some." He doesn't say he *did* all things for all people. He actually did very little for people except what God called him to do: save *some*.

To accomplish that goal, he was willing to give up his personal preferences in dress, customs, and even religious practices. Paul decided, with God's guidance, *what* he was going to do. He let other people determine at times *how* he did it.

We, instead, assert our personality through our clothes, furnishings, and lifestyle. We defend our religious practices far into the night. Then we let other people—families, employers, Christian brothers and sisters, or the latest "How to Improve Yourself" book—set our goals and determine our schedule. Caught between conflicting demands for our commitment and energy, we spend a lot of time just trying to keep people around us happy.

A WISE WOMAN KNOWS:
"Anything you do will make somebody unhappy."

Beth said, "I used to think my stress came from raising four children in the midst of ministry. My husband is a seminary professor, and we often have students and groups in our home. Keeping schedules sorted kept me hopping!"

"Recently I've learned that most of my stress comes from deep inside me. The Hebrew word that we translate 'iniquity' means 'twisted places.' God has showed me that one of my twisted places was being a people pleaser. For years I felt torn by trying to balance husband, kids, and our extended family and friends. Now I'm learning that all I have to do is please the Lord Jesus. I'm concerned about discovering what God wants me to do—and doing only that. Then I don't have to worry when I'm with one person that I ought to be somewhere else or that someone will be unhappy about what I'm doing."

Jesus himself didn't make everybody happy. The Pharisees complained about his doctrine. His mother and brothers got so upset they tried to take him home. His disciples tried to argue him out of what they considered a suicidal trip to Jerusalem. Did that shift Christ from his goals? Of course not! Therefore, at last he could pray, "[Father,] I have brought you glory on earth by completing the work you gave me to do" (John 17:4). Wouldn't that make a marvelous prayer for the end of any life?

Consider for a moment the face of Mother Theresa. Wouldn't it be wonderful to have a face that radiated such joy and confidence because we had accomplished what we were sent to do? But don't buy your plane ticket to Calcutta before you finish this book. We aren't all called to the same ministry, nor must we focus on only one ministry in our lives.

As I have listened to women tell stories about how they have learned to deal with stress, I have come to see that women aren't "get-it-all-together-and-live-with-it-forever" people. Rather, we have seasons in

5

our lives. Each of us has a different set of seasons, and they come in different sequence. They might look something like this: a season of education, a season of work, a season of love, a season of marriage, a season of grief, a season of facing new possibilities, a season of young children, a season of older children, a season of releasing children to adulthood, a season of building, a season of letting go, a season of great productivity, a season of reflection and growth, a season of caring for the world, a season of rest.

Each season has its own stresses—and its own duration. Even while we are accepting the idea that we will *always* be making peanut-butter-and-jelly lunches, grieving for someone lost, or working at one job, that season is passing. We can't predict with any certainty which season will follow, for each of us is unique, created by a loving God who gives us preferences, abilities, and weaknesses and who places us in a harmony of relationships and tasks.

To deal with stress in all our seasons, we must affirm with Ecclesiastes 3:1, "There is a time for everything, and a season for every activity under heaven."

We must see each current season as a part of a larger whole. We must live each season fully, experiencing all its joys and learning all its lessons. Then we must let that season pass and make way for a new one.

The women I interviewed for this book spoke of very different ways they learned to deal with stress in various seasons. As I heard them, I knew that this book dare not *prescribe* (attempt to provide one answer for all women) but could only *describe* —share stories—in the hope that each of us can find answers in these stories for the stress in all our seasons.

In some ways we are alike, of course. We all live in this frenetic era. We all have twenty-four-hour days and seven-day weeks. We all age. We all dream. We all hope. We all can make changes that will reduce the stress in our lives; chapter 6 and the ones that follow it will discuss some of those changes. But first, let's examine what causes our stress—and controls our lives.

EXERCISES

It's time to get out your Bible, pencil, and notebook. Fill your mug with whatever you like best and find a comfortable chair. It may take a while!

What causes stress?

Perhaps your stress is similar to that of some of these women:

Ann: "My mother did all the housework. When I grew up, I still held the ideal that a mother was able to manage the house, but I added a full-time teaching job, two children with a chronic illness that called for significant time and care, and my desire to pursue some of my own activities. That recipe had to spell stress."

Gloria: "This year has been one of incredible stress. My ninety-year-old mother was hospitalized on ten different occasions. It became necessary for us to have her come to live with us, which meant selling our old house and buying one that would accommodate us better. The day after we moved, we were involved in an automobile accident that left me with whiplash injuries. Mother's illness needed nursing care in our home, so I had to find someone to be with her while I was at work. The day after we returned from Virginia for our youngest son's college graduation, Mother died. We held her funeral the day before we left on a long-planned, first trip to Europe. Six weeks after we returned, my husband retired. Stress? Yeah!"

Shirley: "We lost our first child to crib death syndrome when he was six weeks old. When our last child was five, our twenty-year marriage ended in divorce. I had to return to my parents' town, find work to support myself and four children, and build a new life. Talk about stress! If I hadn't come to the Lord, I'd have lost my mind. You can't live with all that and not go crazy."

Donna: "My husband's malignant brain tumor caused a change in our finances and our relationship. We had very different ways of coping, and for a time we felt between us a space we didn't used to have. Also, he had always dreamed of building a business. When he got sick, it failed financially. Having to decide to close up shop in the middle of recuperation was tough on both of us."

Elise: "My youngest daughter and I have been extremely close. Now she's about to go to college. I'm losing my child, a close friend, my primary companion for recreation, and the better part of my wardrobe all at once."

Bonnie: "My physical disability affects both my self-image and my use of time. It means that everything takes so much longer. I have to plan every single movement to conserve energy and time. I also struggle with my singleness. Not as much as I used to, but now and then I see a couple and wonder, 'Why not me, Lord?'"

Or maybe you find yourself on this list of "Common Daily Stressors" handed out to arthritis patients:

too much responsibility
unsolved problems
bad news
threats to self-esteem
no-win situations
uncertainty
computer phone calls
family problems
harassment
time pressure
interruptions
failure
too many commitments
retirement
money
co-workers
job problems
traffic
need to over-achieve
procrastination
friends

Analyze your stress

List *all* your current causes of stress, starting with broad headings such as Too Many Committees, My Husband, My Job. Leave space under each to be more specific—what, exactly, causes stress in each category? List each one.

For example, one for me right now would be "My Children." Under that:
— recent move, no new friends
— summertime: out of school, too hot to be outdoors
— too much television/Nintendo
— frequent interruptions of my work.

Examine your list

I see from my list that it's not my children themselves but their current situation that is causing stress this summer. At other times I could have listed whining, failure to obey, poor sportsmanship, or a poor relationship with a certain teacher—"people" problems we have worked on before.

1. Which of your stresses are caused by situations? Mark them with an *S*.
2. Which of your stresses are caused by people? Mark them with a *P*. Some stresses may be both *S* and *P*.
3. Obviously, we can pray about all our situations. Is your "situation stress" caused by something you can do something else about? If your answer is yes, add a *Y* to the *S* designation (*S-Y*). If your answer is no, add an *N* (*S-N*).
4. Is your "people stress" caused by
   — people who make demands on you? Add a *D* (*P-D*).
   — people you feel responsible for? Add an *R* (*P-R*).
   — people you've overcommitted yourself to? Add an *O* (*P-O*).

Congratulate yourself. Naming the causes of your own stress can be the first step in managing it!

Clear the deck

1. Look at your *S-Y* lists. Circle the situations you can do something about this week. For instance, I see that finding summer activities for my children in their new home is crucial if I'm to have enough stress-free time to finish this book. That involves spending time getting their new rooms organized so they can find games and toys, locating a couple of vacation church school programs, getting library cards, organizing family chore schedules, and researching local pool schedules. Three days invested in their happiness now can free up hours later.
2. What solutions could reduce stress in one or more of your situations? Write them down and plan when you will take those steps. Put the rest of your situation stresses on hold until chapter 6. Except . . .
3. Consider items marked *S-N* , situations about which you can do absolutely nothing but pray. Are you sure you can do nothing about them? You can't change a spouse or co-worker; you can change the way you relate to them, which may change the situation. On the other hand, you really can't do much about rising interest rates on mortgages or your mother's attitude toward your father. If you need help sorting the S-Ns from S-Ys, pray the lovely Serenity Prayer: "God, grant me the serenity to accept the things

I cannot change, the courage to change the things I can, and the wisdom to know the difference."

4. Now do a hard thing: Hand over to God every situation you really can do nothing about. Do it consciously. I recommend praying aloud, not because God needs to hear your voice but because *you* do! It can be as simple a prayer as, "God, I can do absolutely nothing about (name the situation) that has been worrying me and causing stress in my life. I give it to you. Amen."

5. Live out your faith! You've placed those situations in God's hands. Don't permit yourself to worry about them or give them any of your time. Jot down the date you asked God to take care of the situation so you can come back later and see when and how God answered. Because "other people" cause so much stress for women, chapter 5 examines that subject. Save your list of people-related stresses to deal with there.

Who—or what—has control of your life?

Most Christian women—I include myself—would immediately want to reply "Jesus Christ." That's the right answer. But is it real?
Consider your money *

---

* We start with money because most family units spend more than one third of waking time working to pay bills. Chapter 13 will take a closer look at money and its potential for increasing or decreasing our stress.

1. List your last three purchases that cost over fifty dollars. Did you pray about those purchases? Do you use them primarily in God's service?
2. Jot down the price of the place you live in and of the car you drive. At your household's current income, how many hours of work, which means hours of life, will they cost? Are they worth that? Do they give you that much satisfaction or meaning? If Jesus were living your life, would he have chosen them at that price? Why or why not?

Consider your time

1. List everything you remember doing yesterday. Be specific—"dusted, swept, cleaned out a closet, transported three children, made six phone calls" or "made decisions, planned a workshop, sat in boring meeting for two hours, commuted one hour each way to work."
2. Now make yourself feel good. Put a smiley face beside all those things you are glad you did. Be sure to include being nice to that telemarketing person who interrupted you as you were bathing the baby or listening to the employee who popped in for a minute and stayed all afternoon bemoaning her marriage. You may even include tying your garbage securely so the garbage collectors didn't have to smell your rotten chicken bones.
3. How much time did you spend *acting* —taking

13

the initiative in what you did? Mark those items
with an *A* .

4. How much time were you *reacting* to someone
   else's agenda? Mark those items with an *R*.
   After each *R*, list who set your agenda. If what
   you did made them happy, add a +. If what you
   did didn't make them happy or if you are uncertain of their response, add a + or ?.

5. Consider the list one more time. Circle those
   things you think Jesus would have done if he
   had been living your day. Which do you think
   he would not have done? (Remember that
   chores and caring for people are necessary. Jesus
   cooked breakfast on a Galilean beach and
   cleaned up after feeding five thousand. He
   didn't slack off when chores needed to be done!)

   If your whole day was spent on circled *A* items
with smiley faces beside them or if you spent the day
on circled *R* items with smiley faces and so many +
signs that you are satisfied this is the way you want to
live your life, stop reading now and pass this book on
to a friend. Otherwise . . .

Think things over

1. Ask yourself, What does it mean to me to say
   "God is in control of my life"? Write a two- or
   three-sentence statement about what that means
   to you now. Then write what you want it to
   mean in the future.

2. Look at your stress list and your yesterday lists
   again. Who or what is currently in control of
   your life? Who or what sets most of your agenda

or determines how you spend most of your time? Is it one or more other people? Is it a habit? Is it commitments of money or time that have gotten out of control?

3. Ask yourself, If God is in control of my life,
   — did God determine how I spent last Sunday afternoon?
   — did God choose my job?
   — what use does God have for my hobbies?
   — did God assign all the committees I serve on?

Don't panic! You don't need to take immediate, life-changing action in response to any answers you don't like. Just allow yourself to ask the questions and think about them.

4. Read Matthew 22:34—40. What balance does Scripture tell us will result if God controls our lives? What changes will you need to make if you are to know that kind of balance in your life?

Most of us have to admit that God isn't really in control of all of our lives. We do "what we have to do" and "what we want to do"—then we give God the rest of our time and money. A good friend once accused me of giving God credit for running my life so I didn't have to take the blame when things went wrong. That hurt! I'm forced to admit, however, that it's sometimes true. It's far easier to say, "I didn't hear God correctly" or "I don't know why God did that" than to say, "I made the wrong choice."

Ever since Adam and Eve, God has worked in partnership with people, giving us a lot of latitude about how we spend our time and income. Scripture offers guidelines to help us be more effective. Time- and money-management techniques can also help. But the choice is ultimately ours.

"A growing place for me," says Gail, "is to accept that if a day is too full, I've filled it too full. I've accepted too much to do. I'm having to realize that other people and outside forces don't cause my stress. I do. And with God's help, I can control it."

Amen!

Before we talk about how to manage our stress better, however, I want to tell you two stories that have taught me a lot about Christian principles for managing time with much less stress.

CHAPTER TWO

The Master's Model for
Non-Stressed Living

Once upon a time there was a woman who was very busy for God. She worked twenty hours a week as a director of Christian education. She wrote articles for Christian magazines and was part of both a small women's prayer group and a large couples' Bible study. Because she knew God cared for hurting people, she chaired her city's literacy council, served on the board of a home for unwed mothers, chaired its publicity committee, and went to the home one evening a week to befriend the girls. She also knew God cared about justice and hunger, so she served on three hunger committees, volunteered in a local food pantry, taught workshops, edited newsletters for two hunger-relief organizations, and helped coordinate a Christian organization devoted to political advocacy on behalf of the hungry.

Did I mention that her husband directed a city-wide ministry and she sometimes spoke to groups on its behalf?

She did all of that at the same time. What a happy woman she must have been! She was doing so much for God.

Actually she was angry, frustrated, and over-whelmed. No matter how much she did in a day, she always fell into bed knowing she had left important things undone.

Does this sound like your story? It is my own.

That was 1975. My days were filled from morning until long after the sun went down with good works for God. I knew God wanted all those things done and nobody else seemed available. Who would do it all if I didn't?

A WISE WOMAN KNOWS:
*"If you agree to do it,
nobody else will try."*

Have you ever been in that situation? I felt I had to do everything I was doing. But when I woke in the morning I was bone-weary. I snapped at my husband. When I forgot my manners, I even snapped at other people. I sneaked time to pamper myself—read a book for fun, watched a television show in the middle of the day. I felt guilty about doing those things, for I knew I had so many *important* things to do; but some days I just couldn't seem to help myself.

Eventually I developed an addiction to reading trivial books. Not trash, just trivia. Harmless? No addiction is harmless, and I was genuinely addicted.

I went on binges and read seven books in two

days, leaving everything else undone. I read when I felt sick to my stomach for doing it. I begged my husband not to let me read, then I would get out of bed in the middle of the night and go to the front bathroom to read so he couldn't see my light. Finally one evening I took our church youth group to a seminar about alcohol abuse. Reading a list of symptoms of addiction, I had to confess my own. I asked God to deliver me from that particular addiction and packed away all my trivial books.

However, my problem did not get packed away with the books. I simply started watching more television.

Those of you who have been similarly addicted to alcohol, sex, drugs, overeating, or compulsive shopping know what I mean. That kind of addiction comes when the world's demands overwhelm us and we convince ourselves that only *we* can meet our own needs for "fun" in our lives. What we do isn't really fun any more—we know that. But because it was once fun, we do it again and again, hoping this time will be better.

Looking back, it's obvious that something in my life needed to change. At the time, however, I believed that this was the way my life would always be: a seesaw of overwhelming good things to do, then a binge of self-indulgence. I truly believed I was God's servant doing God's work with occasional lapses "to take care of myself."

Finally, one evening I got desperate. The couples' prayer group—all twenty of us—met at our house for dinner and then gathered in the living room. My husband introduced our time of sharing the Lord's Supper with the truth that it is sin to participate in the elements of communion if one is out of charity with brothers and sisters. As I looked around the room, I knew I was out of charity with every person there—simply because they were in my house when I yearned to be alone.

"I'll be back," I whispered to the woman next to me. Slipping out the back door, I headed for my favorite walk next to Tampa Bay. The moon was full over the water, but I scarcely noticed. I was so angry! Since nobody else strolled along the waterfront that evening, I was free to rage aloud.

"Where are the love, joy, and peace you promised if I served you?" I demanded of the Creator of the evening sky. "I'm busy every day all day, and I'm doing it all for you. But there's no love, joy, or peace about it. Is this what serving you is really like?"

In the silence following that cry, I heard the voice of God.

Sometimes I've heard the wisdom of God spoken through Scripture or the words of a friend. I've known the direction of God given through open and closed doors for action. I've felt the nudging of God in my own conscience and mind. That night, I heard the actual voice of God.

It felt as if every pore in my body was an ear, and an enormous sound filled the universe with one startling word: "Rest."

I don't give up easily. "What do you mean 'rest'? I can't rest! Look at everything I have to do. I don't have time to rest. I'm getting seven hours of sleep at the most these days."

Again I heard that enormous, inexorable voice: "Rest."

"Listen one more time," I insisted. "Just look at tomorrow. At seven o'clock in the morning I have a publicity committee meeting at the home for unwed mothers. The whole board meets at eight. By ten o'clock I have to be twenty miles away at a hunger task-force meeting. We get through at noon. All afternoon I meet with the Vacation Bible School committee, and tomorrow night the administrative board meets. Before bed, I'll have to finish an article to meet a Thursday deadline. When am I supposed to rest?"

By this time tears of frustration were streaming down my cheeks, but somewhere deep inside I felt a twinge of hope. If my Boss thought I needed to rest, could that same Boss make it happen? Only one possibility occurred to me: maybe I was about to have a nervous breakdown so I would have to give up everything!

God spoke this time in an idea. "Give up the home for unwed mothers." I knew it was God, because the idea would never have occurred to me. Larry and Flo, members of the group currently meeting in my house, had urged me to serve on that board. It desperately needed me, I was told (and I believed). Could the board get along without me? I had scarcely begun to wonder when I had a not-very-flattering thought. "I don't need you there."

Oh?

"You are doing that for your glory, not mine."

Ouch!

"Well, what about the literacy council?" I asked.

"Serve your term and get off. That will be long enough."

"What about hunger?" I could see responsibilities

21

rolling from my shoulders. Was I to be a free woman at last?

No. Now, filling the universe, the voice spoke two words: "Emphasize it."

A WISE WOMAN KNOWS:
"God doesn't want you busy about everything.
God does want you busy about something.
God even knows what it is."

That was all I heard that evening. I waited around, hoping for more, but all I could hear was the rustle of wind in the palms. Finally, I returned to my house, wondering how I was going to explain this to the group. Especially, what would I say to Larry and Flo?

As soon as I entered my home, I discovered something: God does not work in one person's life without simultaneously working in others' lives to accomplish the same purpose.

When I crept in our back door and started to the living room, Larry was praying—for me! "Lord, we know Patti is stressed out just now. If there is anything I can do to help, show me."

Flo prayed immediately after. "And Lord, we pray for your will to be done in all our lives."

They had not seen me enter, but God had prepared them for what I was about to say. How easily they accepted it. How amazed we all were the next morning when a young man who had far greater publicity skills than I had joined the board. How humbling. How freeing!

The literacy council, too, blossomed after I

resigned. Several people picked up tasks I had been doing and did them better than I had been able to do. Again I was humbled. Again I felt so free.

I wish I could say that since 1975, my life has been free from stress. If I did, would you believe me? You shouldn't. But since that time I've been in a continuing process of learning about God's plans for my life, and I've been trying to concentrate on those plans. Hunger has been the issue I have devoted my volunteer and sometimes professional time to, and I've found that when people call and ask me to work on other issues, it has been easy to say, "That's a really important issue, but my issue is hunger."

I have sometimes been as busy as I was in 1975, but I'm seldom stressed by that busyness. When I am, it's time to retreat and reconsider what I should be doing.

What's the difference between being busy and being stressed? Let's look at our second story, told in Luke 8:40—56.

A rich man's only child became seriously ill. Her father pushed through crowds and urged Jesus to come heal her. Jesus agreed. Surrounded by a crowd, he journeyed toward the house.

Imagine how pressured he must have been by that father. "Hurry, Rabbi, she's dying!"

Imagine how pressured he must have been by the crowd. "What do you think he will do? Jesus, what are you going to do? Can you heal her? Hurry, Rabbi, hurry!" Picture them swarming down the narrow street and jostling bystanders out of the way so Jesus can make his priority appointment on time!

Then a woman comes—not an important woman, not an urgent case. For twelve years she has

23

exhausted her body and her money seeking health. She could wait one more day and see Jesus tomorrow.

Furthermore, she is unclean. Jewish men are forbidden to touch a woman during her menstrual flow, and this woman has hemorrhaged for years. Surely Jesus won't want to deal with her just before entering the home of a leading Pharisee.

She doesn't ask for him to notice her. She just creeps up behind him and touches the hem of his robe.

What would you have done in this situation if you were Jesus?

I know what I would have done—pretended that little interruption hadn't happened. Rushed right on to the "important" thing I had to do.

Jesus stops. He looks around and asks, "Who touched me?"

How frantic that crowd becomes! Luke records particularly the impatience of Peter: "Master [read that in the tone of an adolescent saying "Oh, Mother!"], the people are crowding and pressing against you."

That crowd was stressed. Peter was stressed!

Jesus was not. He was busy but perfectly relaxed.

Watch him stop and scan faces nearest him. Listen to him murmur, almost to himself, "Someone touched me. I know that power has gone out from me."

Then he stands and waits. The crowd fumes. "Why won't he hurry? Doesn't he know the child is deathly ill?"

Finally, trembling, the woman creeps from behind the other people in the crowd and confesses what she has done. Jesus speaks gentle words of comfort: "Daughter, your faith has healed you. Go in peace."

Such a quiet encounter amid such a frantic crowd!

How did Jesus avoid stress in busyness? He spent his life discerning exactly what God wanted him to do. He considered not only the big picture but also the minute-by-minute, day-by-day picture. He was so focused on God that he could discern when an interruption came from God.

He also trusted that if God sent an interruption in the middle of another assignment, God would take care of the assignment until the interruption had been adequately dealt with. Remember the next part of the story, when servants come to inform their master and Jesus that the child had died? Jesus keeps right on walking. "Don't be afraid; just believe, and she will be healed."

Do you want that kind of relaxed confidence as you sort out priorities and choose what to do when? I do!

EXERCISE

Get comfortable and prepare for a few minutes of relaxed thought.

Brother Lawrence, a seventeenth-century lay brother, spent a lifetime "practicing the presence of God"—primarily in a monastery kitchen. He tells how he prayed:

> Sometimes I consider myself there as a stone before a carver, whereof he is to make a statue; presenting myself thus before God, I desire Him to form His perfect image in my soul and make me entirely like Himself.

1. Close your eyes and picture yourself before the throne of God. You are a stone, and he is a carver. Spend five minutes or more asking the Carver to shape you and allowing him to begin to do that.
2. Picture being so in tune with the Spirit of God that life flows smoothly and schedules always work out. Allow yourself to yearn for that kind of tranquility. Turn that yearning into a prayer.
3. Set aside a specific slice of today—even half an hour—to practice God's presence as constantly as you can in whatever you do. Brother Lawrence himself found it hard at first. "One does not become holy all at once," he reminds us.

Once I was teaching at one conference center and my husband, Bob, was teaching forty minutes away. I had agreed to join him for dinner to meet his special friend Chuck. But just as I was about to leave the conference center, a woman came up in obvious pain. What should I do? Bob couldn't be reached by phone; the woman's need was visible. For the first time in my life I winged this prayer: "Lord, take care of Bob and Chuck, please, until we're done here. Don't let them worry about me." Perfectly relaxed, I talked with the woman for over an hour.

When I arrived for dinner—an hour late—Bob and Chuck were just arriving too. "Sorry," they apologized, "we got held up."

This has happened often enough since then for me to know intellectually that when I listen for God's direction in my schedule, I can move at a leisurely pace and still accomplish all that is truly important—sometimes more than I could have imagined!

But I have such trouble living what I know. Far too often I'm still like the crowd—my eye on doing one task efficiently and quickly, resenting interruptions and impatient with delays. Too often I get stressed because I don't listen for God's signals about when to pause and when to get on with the original assignment. One ongoing goal for my life is to get better at hearing

- when to work and when to stop and play with children;
- when to talk on the phone and when to cut it short;
- when to be alone and when to visit a friend instead;
- when to drive on and when to stop to help a fellow traveler.

We will look at those questions, and some ways of arriving at answers, in chapters 6 and following. First, however, we need to consider three barriers that can keep us from even listening for, much less doing, the will of God in our lives.

CHAPTER THREE

Heavy Spirits Are Hard to Carry

Do you know Joanne? Joanne loves her children, her church, her home.

She hates her ex-husband. Talking with Joanne is fun until Walt's name comes up. Somehow it always does. Then her face grows tense, her voice harsh. You want to move away in embarrassment. Joanne went to her doctor with migraine headaches and to a counselor with problems in parenting her children. "Your iron is a bit low," her doctor told her. "Single parenting is hard," her counselor comforted her. She built up her iron and sent her children to college, but Joanne is still bone-tired and depressed. She can't seem to complete tasks or make long-term plans for her life. What could be the matter?

Or maybe you know Mary—a top-notch teacher, a Sunday school teacher, and a choir member. She leads a weekly Bible study. But if you are with Mary for any length of time, you hear about her mother, a domineering, unloving woman who never gave her children respect, attention, or freedom to fail. When Mary's mother came to visit her, members of Mary's Bible study were surprised to meet a spry, cheerful woman who took an interest in their lives and work. They were also surprised to see Mary, usually a gracious hostess, become immature and snappish. What could be the matter?

Sarah is lonely. She wishes she could get close to others but has been disappointed so often that she no longer even tries to make new friends. One former friend betrayed her confidence. Another got married the spring she had promised to go with Sarah to Europe. A third friend—a male—seemed headed for marriage, then veered off. Sarah wasn't surprised. Her own father wasn't very reliable, either. But she wonders sometimes—why aren't people nicer? Why can't they be trusted? What is the matter with everybody?

These are real live people, with real live problems. I changed their names, however, because their real names are Many Women.

What could be the matter?

BARRIER ONE: BLAME AND GUILT

Each of these women faces a barrier to knowing and following God's will. Each is weighed down by rocks of offense: blame and guilt. Each carries hurts inflicted on her by others and guilt for hurts she inflicted in return. In addition, each of them carries anger, resentment, and judgmentalism. Each new offense has been added to the pile until, by now, the loads are enormous. They increase stress, weigh down spirits, color relationships, and prevent these women from becoming all they could be.

Blame and guilt never disappear by themselves. They are removed only by forgiveness and confession. Both are simple. Both are hard.

Forgiveness Heals Blame

The Lord's Prayer teaches that forgiveness is an essential part of the Christian's life: God forgives us *as* (both "while" and "in the manner that") we forgive those who sin against us.

So why don't we do it?

One reason is that we have come to believe that if I can explain *why* I hurt you in terms you can truly understand, you will accept my explanation—and me. Likewise, if you can explain why you hurt me so I can understand, I will accept both the explanation and you. The problem is, *accepting* people as humans who make mistakes is not the same as *forgiving* them. Accepting can be the first step in the process, but that's all it is.

Consider: I may understand why I got the flu from you and that you are a person who is especially susceptible to flu germs. I may even excuse you for giving it to me. That still doesn't cure my flu. Similarly, your understanding why I hurt you and even excusing me won't erase the wounds I inflicted. Genuine wounds and scars need a genuine healing process.

Another reason we don't forgive is that we feel justified in holding on to our grievances. If the other person has not repented, why should we forgive? If they repent, of course, we will deal with them then. But for now, we hang on to our anger. In *Wishful Thinking*, Frederick Buechner says, "Of the Seven Deadly Sins, anger is possibly the most fun. To lick your wounds, to smack your lips over grievances long past . . . is a feast fit for a king."[1]

What we don't realize is that the anger of unforgiveness is like acid destroying its container. We don't notice how blame and guilt slow down everything else we do by wearing out our bodies and consuming our days. We don't know that getting rid of blame and guilt is the first step in relieving our stress.

I learned that very painfully.

When one organization I worked for decided to restructure, the process inflicted a great deal of hurt—especially on long-time employees. I became angry, expecting more humanity than I saw in the new structure and its leaders. Consumed by "a passion for righteousness" (or so I told myself), I found myself unable to sleep at night. When I did, my dreams were angry. Then my nose started to run. Not a drip, but a river that consumed two boxes of tissues a day. I streamed through three final months and with relief left both the job and the city.

My nose kept running.

I visited an allergist but could buy truckloads of tissues for the price of tests he wanted to run. Surely my nose would stop running soon! For another month I dragged on, drippy and dreary.

Then, the Sunday before Christmas, our church's worship service focused on Christ as the bringer of peace and forgiveness. A question nagged my prayers: "Have you forgiven those people?"

(If you don't think God nags, you must be a most obedient disciple. God knows, as most women do, that nagging is telling somebody again what they didn't heed the first time!)

My response to that repeated question was, "Have I forgiven them? Of course not! They hurt not only me but also older men and women who gave their lives to that organization—and they were not the least bit sorry. Why should I forgive them?"

Relentlessly I was hounded in every hymn and reading, even in the sermon, by the words "forgive" and "forgiveness." I found myself facing for the first time the ugliness of my own attitude and anger in the situation. When we got to the Lord's Prayer, I knew I was beaten. I spent that afternoon listing every single person I was angry with and specifically forgiving each offense, then confessing my own nastiness and asking God's forgiveness.

Yes, my nose stopped running. I learned that my nose is God's barometer of stress in my life. For some people it's aching bones, a stutter, or migraine headaches. Thank God for these warning signals that we need to change something in our lives.

I also discovered how much harm unforgiveness—blame—can inflict on bodies and spirits, what a barrier unforgiveness is to getting on with life, and how forgiveness can heal.

A WISE WOMAN KNOWS:
"You should always forgive your enemies.
It will please some and bewilder the rest."[2]

Ways to Forgive

Catherine Marshall discovered yet one more reason to forgive: "I've found this forgiveness business a key to getting prayers answered." [3] Forgiveness not only frees us and the one we have forgiven, it also seems to free up God to relate to us both again!

Marshall tells how David du Plessis, a South African pastor, gave her insights into Matthew 18:18: "Whatever you bind on earth will be bound in heaven, and whatever you loose on earth will be loosed in heaven."

> "For a long time I was puzzled," David told us, "about what 'loosing' and 'binding' meant. Then I found out it means that by hanging on to my judgment of another, I can bind him to the very conditions I'd like to see changed." [4]

Impressed by that insight, Marshall and her husband spent their prayer time for several mornings listing on legal pads their "aughts against any"—anything that caused pain, hurt, or anger to remember. Then they prayed to forgive and release each person from their judgment. In the truest sense of the word, they gave the persons to God. They found themselves freed from bitter feelings about certain people and situations. Shortly they began to see changes in relationships with people they had forgiven.

Not all forgiveness is private. Sometimes it must be a two-way street: We must go to the person who has wronged us to seek reconciliation, not out of a "superior" position (the person wronged), but as one who also has contributed to the pain by carrying grudges, holding on to anger, perhaps gossiping or speaking ill of the other person, or responding to the person with less than full love. This type of forgiveness takes time, but it can result in deeper relationships and spiritual growth for both people.[5]

Frederick Buechner speaks of the healing power of forgiveness: "When somebody you've wronged forgives you, you're spared the dull and self-diminishing throb of a guilty conscience. When you forgive somebody who has wronged you, you're spared the dismal corrosion of bitterness and wounded pride. For both parties, forgiveness means the freedom again to be at peace inside their own skins and to be glad in each other's presence.[6]

Jesus illustrated the highest forgiveness when he spoke from the cross: "Father, forgive them, for they do not know what they are doing" (Luke 23:34). His forgiveness was based on the great truth that it is not our forgiveness that ultimately matters to another, but God's. To return to du Plessis' insight, this type of forgiveness not only releases another from our judgment but also asks God to release that person for all eternity from blame in this matter.

Jesus' cry also reminds us that people are seldom aware of the real consequences of hurtful actions. If a woman knew that her affair with a married man would cause her children to have weak, temporary marriages, would she begin or continue it? If another woman knew that her bitter remarks about her husband would cause his employers to fire him, would she make them? If we knew that criticizing our pastor would weaken our congregation's ministry and cause young Christians to reject Christ's church as backbiting and unloving, would we criticize?

I'm convinced that none of us truly knows the depths of bruises we inflict on others, and other people have no idea of the depth of hurt they inflict on us. Jesus' kind of forgiveness makes us admit the hurt we have caused and release each other eternally.

If our wounds and scars are deep, we may need a trusted pastor or counselor to help us see the extent of our wounds and how the Holy Spirit can help us forgive sins and release sinners. Several authors have written extensively to provide help in choosing a process and a counselor.

Confession Heals Guilt

No matter how hard it is to forgive another person, it's far easier to forgive than it is to confess our own sins. It's even hard for most of us to name them. M. Scott Peck in *People of the Lie* describes people who are skilled at looking righteous while inflicting incredible hurts on others. He suggests that they may have lived with lies for so long that after a while they don't even know they harm others.[7] I suspect we all are, to some extent, people of that same lie, for we live in a society that speaks far more about "false guilt" than the real thing. It's almost impossible to find a good book about confessing our sins—even in a Christian bookstore!

Sadly, the church has been as guilty of repressing guilt as the rest of society. When church hunger committees discuss how to present Western overconsumption as one primary cause of hunger, someone invariably protests, "But, we don't want anybody feeling guilty!" And have you noticed how easily a church-school class of middle-class adults deals with drug abuse or teen immorality rather than with professional ethics in our own businesses or the sins of pride and gluttony at home?

A WISE WOMAN KNOWS:
*"Sometimes the reason you feel guilty
is because you are."*

Not feeling guilty may even persuade us we aren't—not really. I remember once when I got a speeding ticket. Actually, since friends may read this book, I'd better confess that I remember several times when I got speeding tickets. I have a heavy right foot and a secret yearning to drive in the Monte Carlo. (See how hard it is, even when writing about confession, to do it instead of explaining?) That particular day, however, I intended to confess my sin and get on with life.

When I arrived at court, the line was enormous. After waiting half an hour, I found I was in the "not guilty" line. "Where's the 'guilty' line?" I asked.

"Oh, if you were going to plead guilty, you'd just go up to the desk at the front and pay your fine," I was told, "but nobody does that." As I left ten minutes later, fine paid, I couldn't help picturing a similar scene one day in the throne room of heaven.

Ways to Confess

One of the few (and I do mean few!) Christian resources for learning how to confess is the excellent book *How to Repair the Wrong You've Done* by Ken Wilson.[8] Wilson points out that when we have committed a wrong against another person, we may try one of several alternatives to blunt confession: avoid the person, pretend it didn't happen, try to be extra nice, hope the person didn't notice. None of these, unfortunately, has the power to heal wounds and scars. Wilson's book gives practical, wise suggestions for following the scriptural process of confession, repentance, reconciliation, and restitution, if necessary.

How will we know what we should confess? It's so easy to forget our own sins against others. Prayer is one good path to confession. The Holy Spirit, if asked, is happy to show what we need to confess—sometimes when we least expect it.

I remember one retreat when I looked forward to a cozy morning with God and that great psalm of comfort, Psalm 139. I read, "You know when I sit and when I rise."

I heard in my thoughts, "I know how often you sit down and how reluctantly you rise to wait on others or answer the phone to a person in need."

I read, "You discern my going out and my lying down; you are familiar with all my ways."

I heard, "Yes, I know you would rather lie down with a book than go out to the park with your children or help at the soup kitchen. I know the ways you use to avoid leaving your house."

I read, "Before a word is on my tongue, you know it completely, O Lord."

I heard, "Yes, I hear all those words of anger and all that incessant foolish chatter."

Whew! For the first time I understood other language in that psalm: "You hem me in . . . you have laid your hand upon me . . . Where can I go from your Spirit? Where can I flee from your presence?" Words that formerly assured me of the constant loving presence of God became that day a confrontation.

I saw in myself—my energetic, busy self—the old sin of sloth, for I realized for the first time that sloth is not mere laziness but the attitude that I (an avowed servant of Christ) "have a right to" my own time. I saw that sloth is actually idolatry, putting my own self in God's place.

I tell you all this not to confess my sins to you (although the Bible instructs us to do that) but to illustrate that I know from personal experience that if we want to confess, God is willing to help us see what we need to confess.

Christian literature also points toward areas that need confessing. For instance, Wesley's Oxford Club asked questions like

- Do I confidentially pass on to another what was told me in confidence?
- Can I be trusted?
- Is there anybody whom I fear, dislike, disown, criticize, hold a resentment toward or disregard? If so, what am I doing about it?

Oswald Chambers' *My Utmost for His Highest* has an uncanny knack for touching a raw nerve: "Have you 'renounced the hidden things of dishonesty'—the things that your sense of honor will not allow to come to the light? Are you paying your debts from God's standpoint?"[9]

Or you may want to use this confession found in John Baillie's *Diary of Private Prayer*:

A heart hardened with vindictive passions:

An unruly tongue:

A fretful disposition:

An unwillingness to bear the burdens of others:

An undue willingness to let others bear my burdens:

High professions joined to low attainments:

Fine words hiding shabby thoughts:

A friendly face masking a cold heart:

Many neglected opportunities and many uncultivated talents:

Much love and beauty unappreciated and many blessings unacknowledged:

All these I confess to Thee, O God.[10]

EXERCISE

Find a quiet place and uninterrupted time. Get a pencil and a pad of paper. You may want to spread this process over shorter periods for several days or even start now and return later when you have completed the book. If your life has been extremely painful or full of wrongs, you may want to work through a similar process with a trusted counselor.

Forgiving

1. Ask God to reveal to you events that have left you with wounds and scars you still carry: things that still cause you pain, anger, or humiliation. Use one page for each five-year segment of your life and think about one person at a

time, beginning with childhood family members, then current family members, finally branching out to friends, co-workers, and strangers.

2. For each name, write down a word or two to remind you of any incidents you remember. Don't get bogged down in lengthy remembering, and don't write down "always" or "never" items. (My mother never showed me affection. My sister always took my candy.) Ask the Spirit to remind you of *incidents*.

3. When you have completed half an hour of writing, one page of your pad, or one person, go down the list and say aloud, "God, I forgive [name] for [incident]." Speaking aloud can be crucial. Release each person and incident to God.

4. For each incident, confess aloud your own sin in the situation: anger, resentment, keeping it secret, jealousy, bearing a grudge, or whatever the Spirit shows you. Ask God to forgive you for that.

5. Destroy the paper. Burning or flushing creates an effective symbolic gesture!

Confessing

1. Thank God for forgiving your sins and for giving you the power to follow him. State your intention to renounce all wrongdoing, and ask the Holy Spirit to reveal past actions you need to remember.

2. Again think about your life in five-year segments. Beginning with primary relationships

and then others, as before, write down your wrong actions as they come to mind. Don't get sidetracked into daydreaming or lengthy memories.

3. Repent aloud each wrongdoing. Do not explain to God why you did what you did or try to justify it—just ask God to forgive you and give you grace to live as a forgiven person.

4. Star those items that you feel you would like to handle on a person-to-person basis, going to the person and asking for forgiveness. In some cases going to ask forgiveness may not be wise. Ask God in that situation to use your private confession to bless the other person.

5. A long-range strategy may be necessary for extremely damaged relationships. Plan ways to rebuild those.

6. Destroy the paper.

7. Follow up on steps 4 and 5.

Life After

The hardest part about forgiving or confessing is believing we really did it. In the pain of new offenses, old memories come back. We say, "I must not have really forgiven him," or "Maybe God has forgiven me, but I just can't forgive myself."

Concerning the latter, of course you can't! Nobody can forgive herself or himself. God and those we have wronged do the forgiving. We can't guarantee the others, but Scripture promises that God forgives. To speak of forgiving ourselves is arrogant and self-centered, for we want to take for ourselves what belongs to God. An old hymn says, "Just forget about yourself and concentrate on Him." God has promised to forgive, and does.

It is also a matter of Christian discipline to claim that we have forgiven another, God has ratified it, and it is done.

It's not necessary for us to "feel" as if we have confessed or forgiven; it's enough that we have done so. There is one in the universe, however, called the Father of Lies, whose favorite words are, "You didn't really. . . ." One of our faith tasks is to reply, "I did too!"

But—if you try all that and are still haunted by the fear that you have not truly forgiven or confessed, find a counselor who will help you heal those memories. You may need more than one session. The end result—getting rid of barriers so you can get on with life—is worth the time it takes.

CHAPTER FOUR

One Slingshot and Five Smooth Stones

I am convinced that each of us has at least one Philistine in our lives. That Philistine can be a barrier to understanding and carrying out God's plan for us.

Remember the Philistines? Most of us think of them in connection with Samson and Delilah or David and Goliath, but the Philistines are woven through Israel's whole history. Abraham lived with the Philistines for many years. Isaac prospered among them until the jealous Philistines plugged his wells. God told Moses not to lead the Israelites into the Promised Land through the land of the Philistines because, "If [the Israelites] face war, they might change their minds and return to Egypt" (Exod. 13:17). After Joshua's death, several judges, including Samson, struggled against Philistine armies and the influence of Philistine culture and religion. By the time Goliath appeared, Saul had already fought Philistines for years. David fought them well into his kingship. Even in the reign of King Ahaz several generations later, Judah still battled Philistines.

What does that have to do with you and me?

As I live my own life and listen to other women speak of theirs, I find that most of us have one pesky issue that crops up again and again in all our seasons. For one person it is the fear of poverty. She grew up painfully poor. No matter how much she and her husband earned, she worried that one day it would be gone. "Whenever I saw a bag lady, I used to get shivers, afraid that's where I'd end up." At last she thought she had overcome the fear—until her children grew up. Now she wonders if they'll earn enough to live on. "I measure my spiritual growth by how well I deal with that one issue," she ruefully admits.

Another woman wrestles with singleness. "When I was younger, I wanted romance. It was excruciating to see couples holding hands. I got over that, then began to long for companionship. I reached out to friends, found companions, and now I find I yearn for security—somebody who will be there when I get old and sick. My struggles looked different in different times of my life, but it's been the same issue: being single and alone."

My own issue has always been naming God's top priority for my life. My college journals record questions about how much time to study and how much to spend developing relationships. Later I struggled with competing demands of a challenging job, church involvement, and my social life. Still later I wondered which should come first: our children, our marriage, my husband's congregation, or writing?

This book is one fruit of that enduring struggle—and even as I write this paragraph I'm having to decide whether to forge ahead with the chapter or stop a pillow fight and encourage my children as they clean their rooms. What, at this very moment, does God want me to do?

For years I called this my "Philistine issue" merely because it was always there. I felt it was often a barrier to my hearing and doing God's will for my life. Then one day I read this about the Philistines: "These are the nations the Lord left to test all those Israelites who had not experienced any of the wars in Canaan (he did this only to teach warfare to [those] who had not had previous battle experience)" (Judg. 3:1—2).

God *gave* Israel the Philistines to teach warfare and provide a standard against which to measure progress! As I consider my own life and reread old journals, I see that as I mature, I'm dealing better with my own particular Philistine. Like the woman who fears poverty, I can measure my spiritual growth against that one issue.

Take a few minutes to consider your own Philistine. Ask yourself these questions:

1. What one issue have I wrestled with for years?
2. Am I wrestling better now than I was five years ago? Ten years ago? In what ways?
3. What to me would constitute victory over this issue? Record in your notebook the name of your particular Philistine, where you are currently in the struggle, and where you want to be eventually.

BARRIER TWO: HELP!
MY PHILISTINE IS A GIANT!

Once when Israel battled the Philistines, an enormous man came forward. Daily for forty days he strode down a hillside and bellowed a challenge: "Choose a man and have him come down to me. If he is able to fight and kill me, we will become your subjects; but if I overcome him and kill him, you will become our subjects and serve us" (1 Sam. 17:8—9). Israel was paralyzed!

For some women, their recurring life issue is not merely pesky, but debilitating. Daily it saps energy and consumes time and thought, forming a constant barrier between their present and what God would have them to be and do. I call these issues the giant ones. They have names like:

Grief,
Illness,
Addiction,
Recent Divorce,
Mental Illness,
Unemployment,
Depression.

Every day those giants come out onto the hilltops of some lives and roar, "Come fight me. I dare you! Watch me defeat you!"

If you are fighting a giant Philistine, you need to know that this book is not and does not claim to be a manual on How to Battle Giants. But the story of David and his giant Philistine teaches us some principles that may help us in fighting our own giant Philistine—whatever its name and size.

David's Principle 1—
Know You Fight on the Winning Side

David wasn't a better soldier than his brothers. He just believed something they didn't believe: God can give us strength to kill a giant.

Three months before I spoke with Nancy, her husband lost a four-year battle to a degenerative brain disease. She said, "This was a brilliant man, a gentle man, a man with a terrific sense of humor. I grieved as he lost his ability to walk, pick up things from the floor, write, speak clearly. We had been married for thirty years and expected to grow old together. Suddenly, in one day, our life changed. He flew to Mayo Clinic one morning and called me that night with the doctor's diagnosis. They could do nothing for him.

"I remember thinking after I hung up the phone, 'Life is never going to be the same again.' Nobody gets a rehearsal for this. You don't get to practice.

"I was furious with God—banged my fist on many tables. But I learned to thank God that God *is* God. God didn't get bowled over by my fury. Instead, God told me, 'I won't leave you. I'm as sad about this as you are. I grieve with you.' The shared grief of God gets me through my own."

God will fight giants with and for you. David believed it. Nancy believed it. Do you?

PATRICIA H. SPRINKLE

David's Principle 2—
Find a Few Good Stones

Good weapons are crucial in battle. David carefully chose five smooth stones. It only took one of them to kill his particular giant, but he had several in his pouch, just in case. Women who have defeated personal giants point to five resources they have found to be effective weapons: faith in God, people who have fought similar giants, support groups, prayer, and professional help.

Stone 1: Faith in God. Like David, many women are quick to realize that if they had to depend on their own abilities, their attempts to battle giant Philistines would be utterly futile. It is only their faith in God's ability to kill the giant that gives them the courage to go into battle.

When the doctor told Gina he thought she had a fatal skin disease, she faced her giant Philistine: an intense fear of dying. As she waited weeks for the test results to return to her doctor's office, she daily faced her fears—both the real ones and the imagined ones, and they were the worst. She knew from her past that her fears had the potential to choke and incapacitate her as a wife, mother, and nurse. She decided that she could face the giant, but only if God promised to stand with her and give her strength. She found his presence with her through the long weeks, and she also discovered he gave her additional stones for her slingshot: people whose faith she could lean on when hers felt weak, people to embrace her when family members told her they didn't want to hear about her problems, people to pray with her.

Stone 2: People who have fought similar giants. Sometimes we can take comfort from what other people have experienced in similar situations.

> *The toad beneath the harrow knows*
> *Exactly where each tooth-point goes;*
> *The butterfly upon the road*
> *Preaches contentment to that toad.*[1]

This poem in *Rose from Brier*, Amy Carmichael's book of comfort for those who are chronically ill, expresses her frustration at listening to "butterfly" words of comfort from healthy people who had no inkling of her pain, agony, and suffering as she lay in bed for months, recovering from an accident that incapacitated her from her ministry with the Dohnavur fellowship. Amy Carmichael yearned for words from other "toads" who knew the sting of pain.

One of Nancy's stones in facing the loneliness after her husband's death was reading "toad-to-toad" books: "I received a lot of comfort from C. S. Lewis's *A Grief Observed*, written about his wife's death. He says that losing a spouse is like losing your leg. That was *exactly* how I felt. Madeleine L'Engle's *Two-Part Invention* was helpful too after my husband died, although it was too close to our experience for me to read during the process."

"Sandra Simpson LeSourd's *The Compulsive Woman* could have been my own story," another woman declared. "Those shopping binges! She gave me courage to fight to change."

No matter what giant you face, others have faced one with the same name. Some of them have shared their story in print. A visit to a local bookstore or library can help arm you for battle.

Confessing our own weakness to others can also be powerful. One bleak February in Chicago (where February seems to last for twenty weeks in a symphony of gray, black, and blah) someone in our prayer group made the cheery suggestion, "Let's go around and tell what God is doing in our lives these days."

Not taking time to think about what I was saying, I blurted out: "Keeping my usual February depression from becoming suicidal." Then I was horrified. The pastor's wife admitting she got depressed? What would people think?

The next day a new woman in the group called. "I was so glad to hear you say what you did last night. I've been a Christian for nine years, but I still get depressed every winter. I haven't dared to tell any-body—I was afraid they would think I didn't have enough faith. Could we call each other sometimes when things get hard?" That winter I learned again what it is to bear one another's burdens, not merely "somebody else's."

Stone 3: Support groups. At one training event for hunger-action enablers—active, committed people— our meetings invariably started late. "We must have a lot of adult children of alcoholics in this group," one man murmured to me. "Tardiness is something we struggle with." He fished in his pocket and held up a small wooden token. "I just finished my first year in an Adult Children of Alcoholics group."

When I shared his insight with the group, five people knew they had found a new stone for their slingshots. Before the event ended, those five people sought out the man, admitted they faced the same giant, and asked about finding a group for adult children of alcoholics (ACOA). One woman later wrote: "The hunger-response training we got at the workshop was good, but the best thing I got was courage to join an ACOA group and deal with my past."

ACOA is only one of many groups who support one another in giant killing. Other women have said:

- "I didn't understand that I was involved in my husband's drinking problem until I attended Al-Anon."
- "I couldn't have made it through my fight against cancer without my cancer support group."
- "I didn't even believe I had a problem until a friend took me to a group of Women Who Love Too Much. Hearing other people tell their stories was like reading the script of my own relationship."
- "When our baby died, Compassionate Friends got us through. I don't think our marriage could have survived without it."

For almost every giant in the land, we can find a support group to help arm us and stand with us as we battle it. [2]

Stone 4: Prayer. In her lovely novel *A Scent of Water*, Elizabeth Goudge tells of a woman who suffered mental illness all her life. One day she encounters a strange old man who is a fellow sufferer. He gives her three sentence prayers:

> Lord, have mercy.
> Thee I adore.
> Into thy hands.[3]

In my own life, I find that those three little lines—or the Jesus prayer, "Lord Jesus Christ, have mercy on me"—may be all I can pray during a struggle.[4] They are enough.

"Romans 8 has meant a lot to me as I live my days from a wheelchair," says Bonnie. "To know that the Spirit groans with us when we groan and have struggles too deep for words is such a comfort. I get so tired of hassles. Some days I groan a lot. It's nice to know creation and the Holy Spirit are groaning along."

Stone 5: Professional help. Christians are often reluctant to seek professional help to battle giants, yet none of these other "stones" is a substitute for competent professional help when we need it. Sometimes compassionate health and counseling professionals are as necessary to our bodies and minds as qualified mechanics are to our cars.

"We came to one place in our parenting when we knew we didn't have all the answers," Gail admits. "We sought a counselor and took our child for both counseling and prayer. That turned our family situation around."

"I've been so afraid with my new leg braces," says Bonnie. "I knew they weren't quite right, and for two years I was afraid to stand, afraid to walk on my bars, afraid to move from my wheelchair to another chair. I was afraid I'd fall. Finally I called Easter Seals, and they arranged a meeting between me, their physical therapist, the brace company, and my doctor. We are working on the problem together, and I feel as if a huge load has been lifted off me."

David's Principle 3—
Choose a Weapon You Trust

David was offered the king's armor. It was huge and unwieldy, giving Goliath a definite advantage—he had the longer arm.

David considered the matter and said a polite, "No thanks." Instead, he took his own slingshot. It had been effective against lions and bears that had threatened to kill both him and his sheep. He could trust it now.

As women battle giants, it it crucial for us to find counselors, support groups, physicians, psychiatrists, and authors we can trust. Not those who automatically label women "hysterical" or "foolish." Not those who see all women as alike, with the same problems. Not those who automatically prescribe drugs for all pains. Not those who do not know the power of God. Like David, we need to go into battle with trust in our weapons!

One woman spoke of a summer when her teenage

daughter was hospitalized in a juvenile psychiatric unit. "She was assigned a psychiatrist who was openly hostile to our Christian faith. He said in no uncertain terms that she would probably never fully recover, that she was sick because of the way we had brought her up, and that our religion was at the root of all our problems. He was so assertive that after a while we began to doubt ourselves as parents and even as Christians. We had to take a second mortgage on our home to pay his bill so we could go weekly and let him emotionally abuse us.

"For many weeks I prayed, desperate and in incredible pain. One day I received a call from a woman I did not know. She was also a psychiatrist, but she was calling because she was trained as a Stephen minister, someone to befriend others in crisis. For weeks she met with me as a friend. She cared for me, listened to me, and empathized. Through her support we got the strength to believe again in ourselves and our child, and the wisdom to remove our child from the care of that psychiatrist and put her under one who respected our faith and believed in God's power to heal. Gently the new doctor began to work with our family. Almost immediately our daughter began to get better."

Another woman told about going to a counselor after her husband had committed adultery. "She may have been a good counselor for some people, but not for a person of faith. She told me I needed to look after my own interests, get my life together, and leave him. Not once did she suggest that I was partly responsible for what had happened, although I knew in my heart I was, nor did she ever encourage me to try to work with my husband to put our marriage back together. Thank God we had some friends who were able to steer me to another counselor, one who prayed with me and then counseled with both of us. Our family is stronger now than it has been for years, but if I had stayed with the first counselor, our marriage would have been dissolved."

The world is full of people who want to offer us "Saul's armor" solutions with which to battle our giants: the latest in the world's pills, ideas, diets, and answers. Thank God there are also persons with genuine and proven compassion, wisdom, and training who can offer solutions that truly kill giants once and for all. If you are uncertain about who might help with your particular giant, ask pastors in your community to recommend a support group, Christian physician or counselor, or call the national offices of professional organizations of Christian counselors and psychiatrists for a referral. Some such organizations are: The American Association of Pastoral Counselors (703-385-6967); and The Samaritan Institute (303-691-0144). For suggestions of a congregation near you with laypersons trained in supportive ministry, call Stephen Ministries (314-645-5511).

Like David, when we go into battle with giants, we need weapons we can trust!

EXERCISE

It's possible that you've read this chapter, admitted that you have a giant in your life, but decided you would prefer to ignore your giant for now while you use this book to help you battle smaller Philistines first. If so, please read 1 Samuel 17 again.

Once Goliath entered the field, all other warfare was put on hold. A giant is a major barrier! Therefore, until you have overcome your personal giant, no book on earth can help you get the rest of your life in order.

What will you do *today* to get ready for your battle? A few suggestions:

1. The first—and often hardest step—in killing a giant is naming it. Write down the name of your giant and a sentence or two describing how the giant is preventing you from being all God meant you to be.

2. Pray, asking God to help you battle this giant to its death in your life.

3. Commit yourself to the battle. Sometimes it helps to confide in a trusted friend and ask the friend to hold you accountable. Set a date to meet with the friend to discuss your progress.

4. Take one step today toward collecting your stones: buy and read one book by someone who has battled a similar giant, call and make an appointment with a professional, or commit yourself to attending the meeting of a support group in the next week.

CHAPTER FIVE

I Do It All for You, Dear!

The greatest barrier to women's accomplishing our own life goals is the time we spend helping *other people* meet theirs.

I sometimes think that the parable of the three stewards (Matt. 25:14—30) should have included a fourth character—a "stewardess"—who comes back to the master with the original talents in her pocket. "I was going to invest them on Monday, but little Mikey got the flu. On Tuesday a friend's marriage fell apart. On Wednesday my mother needed me to take her shopping. Thursday was my day to drive Meals on Wheels, and Friday my boss had an emergency, so I had to work late. If you'd been gone just a little longer, I'd have invested those talents and made more profit than anybody."

A WISE WOMAN KNOWS:
*"If you don't decide how to spend your life,
somebody else will decide for you."*

In a perfect world, of course, Jesus would have awarded her the whole pot for her selfless behavior. Since he did not, I fear we must conclude he meant what the parable said: Stewardesses, like stewards, are rewarded not by how much good we do, but by how well we obey our Creator's orders.

BARRIER THREE: MEETING OTHER PEOPLE'S NEEDS

It's hard to obey God's orders, however, when we define ourselves primarily by our relationship to somebody else. Have you ever noticed how often women are introduced as somebody else's wife, mother, daughter, or employee? Men are defined by their own employment, women by our connections!

A good bit of that is our own fault. I'm often amazed at how we women expand Scripture. For instance, we broaden Ephesians 5:22, "submit to your husband," to include submitting our own callings, desires, and needs to those of *any* man, woman, or child who demands some of our time. Then we justify that behavior with Romans 12:1, "Offer your bodies as living sacrifices"—forgetting that what Paul actually said was, "living sacrifices, holy and *pleasing to God*" (italics added).

Beth tells how that worked in her life. "Since college I've had life goals. I've re-evaluated them from time to time, but they've stayed pretty much the same. One is to know God, not be a mediocre Christian. Another is to discover who I am in relation to Jesus. The third and fourth are to have a close marriage and to invest myself in my family.

"But recently I got a hard lesson. When we sent our oldest off to college and the youngest to first grade the same fall, I thought I would die. I discovered that I had made mothering an end in itself. One day in a parking lot God revealed to me that I am essentially and existentially alone. I realized that my family is a gift, not a given. One traffic accident could take them all from me—and then who would I be? I now know that Jesus, not my family, has to become the center of my life."

Why Do We Wrap Ourselves in Others' Needs?

Sometimes we genuinely think we should. Poor or partial interpretations of Scripture have convinced us that women have been created by God primarily to take care of other people. The truth, of course, is that both male and female Christians have been called to serve others—but *only* after obeying the first and greatest commandment: "Love the Lord your God with all your heart and with all your soul and with all your mind" (Matt. 22:37). Whenever the needs or demands of others get in the way of what we feel God calls us to do or be, we need to pray in order to discern exactly how to resolve that conflict.

Unfortunately, most of us don't let the needs of others consume us for wholly spiritual reasons.

Ann, whose daughters both developed juvenile diabetes before they were three years old, said, "I had low expectations of help from my children, and was willing to spend money and most of my free time taxiing them to dance classes, art lessons, cheerleading, horseback riding, piano lessons, Brownies, Girl Scouts, and choir because I thought I could compensate to some degree for the shots, food restrictions, blood and urine tests, and emergency rooms that were often part of their childhoods. So I taught all day, graded papers in parking lots, did most of the cooking, cleaning, laundry, and dishes, and was exhausted much of the time. I see the same thing now in other friends whose children have been hurt by divorce. We excuse our children from helping at home to make up for their living in a less-than-perfect world."

Betty identified another reason why we "do it all" for those around us. "For me, it was an issue of control. I tried to control my husband, children, and others within the sphere of my environment in order to control that environment. I thought I needed to control them in order to control my own life. I couldn't nap, for instance, because I worried, 'What if that serviceman came? Could the kids tell him what to do?' God finally had to remind me that I'm not called on to be God, who sleeps neither day nor night. I had to learn to lay down my compulsion to control. Ultimately we can control only our own lives; we can discipline only our own lives."

Years ago a poet read this in a writers' group I attended. It spoke to me that night and has haunted me ever since.

Little Red Wagon
by Kimberlee Ann Burdick

During her tenth summer
she loved playing mommy to baby sister.
Each day baby climbed into the little red wagon
pleading for a ride.

Because she loved the cargo
little mommy pulled the wagon.

Looking ahead, she pulled with strong fervor.
After all, baby needed mommy!
Over the summer, it became routine.
Little mommy had found her call.

Summer passed
as did the years.

Because she loved pulling the wagon,
little mommy accepted the cargo.

Looking ahead, she pulled with tired determina-
tion.
After all, this was her duty!
But it became a drudgery
and little mommy was exhausted.

Glancing behind, she groaned,
"How did you ALL get in my wagon?
I can't keep pulling much longer."
(Baby sister had been joined by daddy
and mommy and friends and even some
strangers!)

Looking bewildered, they all screamed,
"Stop your damned pulling and we'll get out!" [1]

Notice that at first the little mommy pulled the
wagon because she loved the *cargo*. Then she
accepted the cargo because she loved the *pulling*.

Each time I read that, something inside me says, "Ouch!"

Sometimes we pull others because we fear they'll never be able to pull themselves. After Mary Gene's husband asked for a divorce, he developed a debilitating illness with a long recovery period. She agreed to postpone the divorce until she had nursed him through. "My priest at the time spoke of my 'fire-bucket behavior' and suggested I let my husband suffer the consequences of his own decisions. He was right. But I find myself often slipping back, having to fight every day not to believe I have to rescue the world or the people I love from the consequences of their actions."

Sometimes we even help others when they neither want nor need that much help! A dream showed me I did that frequently. I don't usually tell my dreams, but this one may sound familiar to someone:

I was biking past a restaurant and saw two friends finishing lunch inside. They invited me to join them. Then they suggested we visit the gift shop next door. I didn't want to (I hate to browse), but since they did, I went. I searched for something—anything—to buy, to redeem the time. Finally, I found a pair of earrings for one dollar—all the money I had. As we were leaving, I noticed that the earrings were rusty. "I need to exchange these," I exclaimed. But my friends were in a hurry and had to leave. I spent the rest of my dream trying to find something else for which I could exchange those earrings.

In discussing that dream with Bob later, we saw that I often had "rusty earrings" in my life: places I agreed to go or tasks I agreed to do because somebody else suggested it. Because I never checked to see how important the tasks were to the ones who suggested them, I often got left doing the lion's share of work while the others drifted away to something they valued far more.

Does that sound familiar to any of you? Since having that dream, I ask the person or group asking me to take on a new activity, "How important is this to you on a scale of one to ten? How committed are you to this task?" If it doesn't matter to them, I certainly don't intend to spend a lot of my time on it either. When Bob and I discuss whether or not we will take on certain responsibilities as a couple, we sometimes agree, "Sounds like a rusty earring."

Helen has learned a similar lesson. "When people tell me a job won't take much time, I now ask them exactly what they think it will entail—and who will do the detail work. If people think a job is important enough to ask you to do it, it will probably take a lot longer than they first tell you it will!"

How to Live With Other People Without Wearing Out in the Process

Obviously we are going to continue to live with, love, and serve other people. But we can take some steps to relieve the stress serving can bring on us.
Just Say No. I start with this one because saying no is the hardest. It involves admitting we are not indispensable, that others can indeed do some things for themselves, and that people can and do get out and walk alone if we stop pulling. It involves convincing ourselves that what *we* feel called to do (or even just

want to do) may be as important as what others ask us to do. It may even result in something very scary for some of us: free time.

Share the Family Load. As I interviewed for this book, I discovered that some women are doing too much because their husbands and children are doing too little! Many children today have never been taught to mop a floor, sort laundry, or cook a nutritious meal, and have no regular chores. One friend, hearing that her daughter was admitted to Yale, groaned, "Only nine months to teach her everything she needs to know to live on her own."

Some mothers of grown children I interviewed said wistfully, "I wish I'd expected more from my children when they were at home. It would have made things easier for all of us, and prepared them better for adulthood." Inspired by their regrets, I wrote a companion book to this one, entitled *Do I Have To? What to do About Children Who Do Too Little Around the House* (Zondervan, 1993). Research for that book convinced me that failure to give children regular household tasks does both parents and children a great disservice. Children deserve to learn how to take care of their own basic needs before adulthood. They need to learn to function as a member of a family team. And they need to learn responsibility and accountability before they apply for their first job.

On the other hands, a mother whose family shares household chores eventually has less stress.

I say "eventually," because a mother may experience increased stress when children first start doing chores. They need to be trained and persistently motivated at the beginning. Furthermore, most women are used to thinking of the house as "mine," not "ours," and want it cleaned "my" way instead of "our" way. When we give up that need to control, however, and share the load, a good bit of stress disappears. It's nice to cook and do dishes only on your own nights, and to clean one fourth of a house and know your work is done.

Negotiate and Reciprocate. In our family, Bob likes football, and I like plays. We used to do neither since we each felt reluctant to spend time and money on something primarily for our own pleasure. And we secretly resented the other for occasional games or plays. Now each fall we decide how many football games and how many plays we'll see. Sometimes we go together; sometimes we take a friend instead. Each of us gets to do something we value while providing a chance for the other to do something valuable too.

Likewise, children can learn to swap favors. If I drive my boys to baseball practice, for instance, I may ask them to prepare dinner later so I can finish a chapter. Beth says, "Our children have been taught that our family is in ministry together. We entertain everybody's friends, so we all pitch in to make that happen: clean together, prepare together, entertain together. We stress a family sense of commitment. When we clean, the kids grumble sometimes, but we stress a good attitude."

Negotiation also works when we find we are resisting a certain task. A real peeve of mine is people who leave laundry in the dryer. Bob's peeve is people who leave clean dishes in the dishwasher. So, in the providence of God, we married our peeves. For years we nagged each other, until one evening when I was pulling wrinkled sheets out of the dryer just as he opened the dishwasher and bellowed, "Who left these dishes in here?"

I shouted back, "The person who won't say a word about these sheets if you don't mention those dishes again!" We sat down and made a pact: We won't try to change the other. We won't try to change ourselves. We will live with our differences and take out what we hate to see left in. Nothing changed; everything changed.

Negotiating does involve admitting we can't have everything our way. For me, it was deciding that if Bob really likes our bedroom better with fifty dirty socks under his dresser, he should be permitted to have it that way. For him, it was agreeing that I wasn't "supposed" to pick up socks from under his dresser.

In a workshop I attended, a woman complained that her husband does absolutely nothing around the house. "What do you want him to do?" somebody asked her.

"Well, since I clean the house, I want him to do the yard. But he won't. He wants to hire it done. I think that's extravagant, so I end up doing it."

Can you see how her "doing" the yardwork was also an attempt to control her husband? The group caught on to that immediately. Since her husband had money to hire the lawn done, it was his right to decide whether to do the work or pay for it to be done.

That raises another question: Is it fair to take "family" money to pay for things that only *we* want done, like extra baby-sitting or an occasional housecleaning service? I'm a firm believer in "his," "hers," and "ours" bank accounts. I know some families manage amicably with one account, but we find that individual, monthly discretionary allowances reduce stress and let us indulge ourselves and each other.

I have written as if negotiation and reciprocation occur only at home. That is far from the case. In my experience, however, we are better at sharing overloads and dividing tasks according to preference and ability at our workplaces than we are in our homes. If this is not the case for you, consider how you can begin to negotiate and reciprocate where you work.

Sometimes neighbors, friends, and elderly parents can demand a good bit of time. One woman I know has learned to reciprocate and negotiate with her mother. "If I take you for a drive this afternoon, I want you to come to our house and be with the children next Tuesday so I can go to the library and read in peace for an hour." How often do we "do it all" for some people because we fail to see the valid, important things they can do in return?

Barter or Hire. Most of us don't have funds to hire full-time housekeepers, chauffeurs, and lawn services. Most mothers, however, are well aware of the benefits of carpools or swapped mornings of childcare. As I speak with women who feel trapped by the demands of small children, elderly parents, too much to do at home or work, or too little money, I find that they often haven't fully explored other possibilities for bartering or hiring care that can free them for at least some time each week. Hiring involves paying, of course. Bartering involves swapping something you can make or do for someone else's time and ability.

Have you swapped weekends with another couple, watching each other's children in exchange for a getaway of your own? A single friend of mine often swaps apartments with friends in other cities, providing each with an inexpensive base for a vacation week.

Have you hired a young teenager to watch children or sit with an elderly parent for a few hours each summer week, so you can work on a big project? My youngest sitter was ten. She amused my children, then five and two, each morning one summer while I sat on the front porch and wrote a book.

Have you considered hiring a teenager to clean your house a few hours each week after school? Four hours after school can do wonders for your morale and his or her bank account.

In one neighborhood, women cleaned each other's houses for equal pay, instead of cleaning their own.

Have you tried to find church people who could sit with elderly, housebound adults a few hours a week in exchange for something you do well—baking bread, mending, or driving?

In your office, have you considered what tasks could be done by bringing your elementary-school children or young teenagers in after school, paying them with tickets to movies, gift certificates, or video rentals rather than a wage? I have seen children sort files, file records, pack boxes, make copies, and answer phones. And at that age, routine office chores look important and fun.

Confront. Bob and I ran into our neighbors and a couple we did not know at the polls. "Come, meet these people," the husband said to their companions. "They're good neighbors."

"Sure are," the wife agreed. "They taught us how to fight."

That was not what I had hoped she would say. I have since decided, however, that that was not a bad thing for them to have learned. Women often avoid conflict, thinking it's not ladylike to fight. But fighting fair—confronting one another, sticking to one topic, making sure each person gets a fair chance to say "I want" or "I need" and working for a mutually satisfactory outcome to conflict—is an important part of any relationship.

EXERCISE

People who cause you stress

1. Go back to the stress list you made in the exercise to chapter 1. Consider those stresses on your *P-D* list, people who make demands on you. Do you see places where you already have the courage and are willing to take the power to make some changes? For instance, are there people who truly should be told "no" the next time they ask for your time? Will you do that?

2. Are there people who are demanding large chunks of your time lamenting situations they don't plan to change? Can you tell them, lovingly but firmly, that they need more help than you can give—perhaps even suggest a support group or counselor for them—but let them know you are neither capable nor willing to help them perpetuate their problem?

3. Consider your *P-R* list, people you feel responsible

for. Is there someone you could share that
responsibility with (e.g., family members, community service organizations)? Are you perhaps
taking more responsibility than you need to?
What changes can you make in any of those situations?

4. If one of your people issues is a "giant," such as
an alcoholic spouse or a family member who
requires constant care, do you need to find a
support group for yourself? What one step will
you take today to make that happen?

5. Save your *P-O* list (people to whom you are
overcommitted) until we set life goals in the
next chapter.

People who can help reduce your stress

1. List what causes the most stress in your most
intimate relationships (e.g., what are most fights
about?). Ask yourself:
   — Am I acting like a "fire-bucket brigade," trying to save someone from the consequences
of his or her own actions?
   — Am I pulling a wagon for someone who
could be walking?
   — Am I trying to compensate for something in
his or her life?
   — Am I helping this person learn to stand
alone?
   — Am I permitting this person choice about his
or her issues?

2. Consider the way you normally relate to other
people. What stress-producing tasks and situa-

tions could you negotiate or reciprocate with someone else?

3. What tasks could you hire or barter in exchange of services to get done?

Other people in our lives can be bothers or blessings. They can be barriers to finding out what God wants us to do and doing it, or they can be partners in the search and the process. Ultimately, whether they are barriers or blessings depends on what we permit them to be.

CHAPTER SIX

Picture a Perfect You

A godly old woman was once asked, "Do you ever worry that when you get to heaven, God will ask, 'Why were you not more like St. Catherine or St. Joan?'"

"Ah, no," she sighed. "I worry that when I get to heaven, God will ask, 'Why were you not more like yourself?'"

Dag Hammerskjöld writes,

> At every moment you choose yourself. But do you choose *your* self? Body and soul contain a thousand possibilities out of which you can build many Is. But in only one of them is there a congruence of the elector and the elected. Only one—which you will never find until you have excluded all those superficial and fleeting possibilities of being and doing with which you toy . . . and which hinder you from [discovering] the talent entrusted to you which is your I. [1]

Have you ever pictured a perfect you? If not, take a few minutes now and imagine the following scene: You are seated at a table. A woman comes into the room and sits across from you. You meet, for the first time, Who You Really Could Be. She is exactly your age and is living your life.

What does she look like? What is she doing with her life? How is she maturing as she ages? What tone of voice does she use? How does she respond to interruptions? In what ways is she powerful or gentle, tough or soft?

Now the whammy question: How does she differ from you now?

Okay, so first you noticed she weighs twenty pounds less, has fewer wrinkles, and better-cut hair. But what else do you see?

What will she accomplish in her life next year? What emotional tone does she bring into a room? What crazy dreams does she have? Who or what do you see when you look into her eyes? What gives her the most joy?

Dreaming about what we could be and do is something few of us take time to do. Yet both Scripture and psychology tell us that we become what we focus our thoughts on. Some exercises at the end of this chapter will help you dream about the person you want to become. This can be the most important step in reducing the stress in our lives.

A WISE WOMAN KNOWS:
*"If you know what you want to be and do,
you'll also know what you don't have to be or do."*

Many of us, especially those of us with super-woman tendencies, live at the mercy of old habits, others' demands, desires to escape, or voices that say we "should" be doing this or that. Deciding what new habits to develop, whom we should serve, how, and what else we truly should be doing frees us from those forces. It also frees us from thinking that the most important thing about us is what we *do*.

In *Letters to an American Lady*, C. S. Lewis warns, "Don't be too easily convinced that God really wants you to do all sorts of work you needn't do. . . . Remember that a belief in the virtues of doing for doing's sake is characteristically feminine, characteristically American, and characteristically modern."[2]

Ann said, "In college I had a goal to become a mature Christian woman. But in the next fifteen years my goals shifted. I wanted to be a successful super-mom, a great teacher, a fabulous wife. All these involved a lot of *doing*, so I measured myself by how well I did. Not until we had a family crisis with one of our teenagers did I get back to my original goal. Now my goals are not to *do*, but to *be*: to be united with the Holy Spirit, allowing my mind to be filled with the mind of Christ; to be free of anxiety, always trusting God to care for me and my family; to be used continually to bring Jesus into the environment in a winsome way; to experience continually the joy and peace that God offers; and to be a walking example of all that."

GIVING WINGS TO OUR DREAMS

In order to move from what we dream about being and doing toward really being and doing it, we need to do two things: set goals for our lives, and plan how to achieve those goals.

Already I can hear somebody voicing one of three objections:

"I don't have time to set goals and plan!"

"Setting goals and planning are far too complicated!"

"Setting goals and planning isn't Christian! We should trust God for everything."

I Don't Have Time for Setting Goals and Planning

To the first I say, if you are very busy and under stress, you can't afford *not* to set goals and plan. I've been where you are. For years I looked for those few golden tips that would put my life in order. I had periods of great efficiency, balanced with periods of guilt because I had let everything fall apart. (Have you ever noticed that some books are written so that if you succeed, they get the credit and if you fail, you get the blame?) Once a year, usually around my birthday or New Year's Day, I would look at past months and know I had done very little that really mattered to me or to God. Unless we have visionary, overarching goals and plans that can help us reach those goals, mere achievements can leave us feeling unsatisfied.

A WISE WOMAN KNOWS:
*"If you don't know where you want to go,
you'll never know whether you get there."*

Goal Setting and Planning Are Too Complicated

To those who think goal setting and planning are complicated, let me suggest that most of us work with goals, plans, and time-management skills every day of our lives. Consider, for instance, making an omelette:

Swiss Cheese Omelette

Beat egg, add salt, pepper, and 1 tsp. water. Pour onto buttered griddle over medium heat. Cook slowly until egg sets. Sprinkle grated Swiss cheese on one side; fold other side over to cover. Let cheese melt. Remove to plate. Eat.

The *goal* —what we want to do—is to make an edible omelette. The *plans* include gathering ingredients, beating the egg, grating the cheese, melting the butter, and so on. *Time-management skills* are involved in deciding when to do what.

A novice cook may butter the pan and turn on the heat, then go looking for an egg. By the time she has beaten the egg, the butter is too brown. By the time she has found the cheese and the grater, the egg is burned. It's almost impossible to cook a good omelette—or get through a woman's day—without setting goals, making plans, and using time-management skills!

Is It Christian to Set Goals and Plan?

This last objection to planning deserves a longer answer, because it too often blocks women from taking charge of their lives. By "taking charge" I do not mean that we seize authority that belongs to God but that we begin to seek God's will for our lives and make plans to move in that direction instead of letting other people set our days' agenda.

But is it "Christian" to plan? Aren't we supposed to "wait on the Lord," and "listen to the Spirit" for guidance? Yes—and no. Scriptural examples show that we wait on the Lord for an idea of what we are supposed to do, then we plan how to do it.

Most of us do this already in a small measure. For example, once we decide it's in God's will that we get married, eat, work, or take time off, we go ahead and plan our weddings, menus, office procedures, and vacations. The only important event we are content to muddle through without plans is life itself!

We may even quote, "Take no thought for your life" (Matt. 6:25 KJV) to prove our point. But Jesus was talking about worrying, not planning. He said we are not to worry about material needs, for God supplies those *as we work toward the goal*: seeking God's kingdom and righteousness (Matt. 6:33). Doesn't *that* entail some planning?

Jesus seems to have thought so. He compared deciding to follow him with the process of building a tower or making war—situations requiring detailed planning (Luke 14:28—33). His parables praise wise servants who plan to welcome the master home (Luke 12:35—38) and a crafty steward who plans his future after his master fires him (Luke 16:1—9). Perhaps the longest "pro-planning" chapter in the Gospels is Matthew 25, which reveals three examples in which poor planning resulted in disaster: the story of five foolish women whose poor planning caused them to miss a wedding; the story of a foolish steward whose poor financial planning ruined him; the story of a final judgment day when nations are divided like sheep from goats, based on whether or not they fed the hungry, housed the homeless, clothed the needy, visited the sick and imprisoned—all of which require planning to accomplish.

When the Spirit told Christ the time was ripe, he also *planned* to go to the Cross: "As the time approached for him to be taken up to heaven, [he] resolutely set out for Jerusalem" (Luke 9:51).

Jesus is not the only one in Scripture who heard the Spirit say, "Here's the job, this is the season" and immediately began to plan ways to accomplish a goal. Nehemiah, called to restore Jerusalem's walls, planned carefully enough to give his king precise lists of what he needed. Esther, called to stop the imminent destruction of all Jews in Persia, fasted and prayed for three days, then executed a carefully planned campaign to persuade her husband to reverse the order. Naomi, eager to become a grandmother, illustrates delightful planning in Ruth 2 and 3. (Or did you think Boaz and Ruth met in that wheat field by accident?) David's battle strategies, the Apostle's appointing of deacons, Paul's missionary journeys—all were carefully planned. If setting goals and making plans to achieve them were important for those people of God, are they any less necessary for us?

Granted, we must hold our plans lightly, and prayer-fully, in case the Holy Spirit chooses to alter them. In Acts 16, Paul was on his way to Bithynia when the Spirit sent him to Macedonia instead. Note, however, that Paul was not sitting around awaiting instructions when the Spirit intervened. Paul planned to go to Bithynia, then planned how to get to Macedonia.

As I interviewed women for this book, few of them had sat down and written purpose statements for their lives. "We didn't used to do that," one said wryly. But as we spoke, most of them could now look back and say what goals they have been working toward out of a prayerfully developed vision.

Maxine, Helen, and Gail want "to serve others, to make a real difference in people's lives and situations." Beth wants "to know God deeply—not be a mediocre Christian—and to find out who I am in him." Shirley wants to "leave my children with a good relationship to me and to the Lord."

On a different plane, Shirley also wants a fishing camp where she can fish with her grandchildren. Bonnie envisions a perfect retirement center where she can shop, wander outside, attend events, and visit others in her wheelchair. Elise and Beth want to invest themselves in other women, helping them grow strong and capable. Maxine wants to go around the world. "That's our pre-nuptial agreement. I was working my way around the world when I met Bud. We got to talking about getting married, and I said, 'I can't get married—I'm going around the world!' Bud promised he would take me, and he's been doing it ever since." They had just come back from Alaska when we spoke.

Each of these visions was suited to the personality, abilities, and inclinations of the women who held them. We are unique. Can we say that often enough? God has created women unique so that we can be—and do—unique things.

As we also have said before, we live in seasons. Therefore we may work toward each of our goals in different ways in different seasons. Or we may focus on one goal during a particular season.

Betty said, "My ultimate goal is to be God's person, dedicated totally to knowing and serving him. But in my prayer life, God has revealed times and seasons for other goals. It was as if a spotlight came and focused on me.

"At one time parenting was it. We had recently moved to Britain, and our children were young at the time. My husband needed to return to the States frequently to meet previously made commitments. Things were in such an upheaval that I realized I had to be an absolute anchor for my children. My focus was to provide security for them.

"At a later season I had another primary commitment: to establish a music business that would provide a good bit of income for the Community of Celebration, the religious community in which my husband and I both lived and worked. God kept giving me ideas and visions for how that could work. It was the key to our financial security in those days, and God showed me how to make it happen.

"During a period when the community was planning to relocate and we had come back to the United States as forerunners, my husband had a heart attack. I had been centered on music, our family, and the community for several years, but at that time God indicated I was to be involved in outreach for a season. For three to four years I traveled quite a lot, keeping networks open.

"Later God centered me on the maturing life of our community—being available to the community and to our growing ministry within our denomination."

"How do you know if you are doing what God wants you to do?" I asked.

She smiled. "God gives a discernible peace in the context of life, a peaceable presence along the way. Ideas are given, doors are opened. God gives forward movement."

God's forward movement. That's what we are talking about—taking God seriously in Jeremiah 29:11, "I know the plans I have for you" and moving forward from there.

EXERCISE

Curl up with your paper, pen, and Bible again. Give yourself plenty of time to reflect, study Scripture, and write.

A WISE WOMAN KNOWS:
*"Planning involves praying,
thinking, and writing!"*

What do you want to do with the rest of your life?

Although your immediate response may be, "I just want to get through my present stage," think ahead toward the end of your life. What do you want to accomplish? What will you regret never having been or done?

What are you currently doing?

1. List everything you currently do with your time in a year. List each committee separately and indicate if you have an office that requires additional time beyond meetings. List pieces of large jobs separately. For example, instead of "mother two children," list "volunteer in school library; drive to baseball, ballet, orthodontist; pack lunches; arrange family recreational outings." Instead of "work," list different tasks related to your job. The purpose of this list is to get down on paper some idea of how you spend all your hours each month, so the more detailed you are now, the easier your planning will be later.

2. Next to each item, list how many hours you estimate you spend doing that in a month's time.

3. Set priorities: prayerfully rank each item A (very important for me to do), B (less important for me to do), and C (not important for me to do). As you rank, remember that you are seeking what is important for you to be doing. Many worthwhile tasks need doing. The important thing is to give up the notion that God wants you personally to do everything that is worthwhile!

A WISE WOMAN KNOWS:
"The greatest enemy of the best you can do
is not the worst you can do,
but the almost-best."

If you aren't accustomed to listening for God, these sources of God-given wisdom may help you decide what you can, or even should, eliminate.

— What are God's priorities? Look again at Matthew 6:33 and Matthew 22:36—40. How does each thing you are doing measure up to those standards?

—What do you do well? Not so well? Your abilities are God given. Honor them!

—What are your deepest longings? Most of those are God given. Pray to discern which ones are biblical and honor them.

— What gives you joy? Maybe you're a whiz at math, but you hate it. Trust your sense of what gives you joy.

4. Eliminate the garbage. All of us have to do some things we do not value, but can you already see ways to get rid of the most time-consuming or least valuable ones? Ideas: Stop! Share the Work! Find someone else to do it! Plan how you will get rid of each. Follow through!

FROM ORIENTAL PHILOSOPHER
LIN YU TANG:
"Besides the noble art of getting things done,
there is the noble art of leaving things undone."

Consider your life by categories

1. At this point, relist your A items by categories, using as headings various arenas in which you spend your life. For instance, I group my own under Personal Growth, Family, Church, Community, Writing, Hunger, and House/Yard.
2. Ask yourself: Is there something I wish I were doing but it doesn't appear here as a category— perhaps personal faith development, recreation, or travel? Add a category—you are about to begin to dream!
3. Do you need a category to help you deal with a personal Philistine issue? Add it as well.

Draft a life-goal statement

1. For each category of your life, prayerfully consider what one or two things you want to accomplish in your lifetime. Write a life-goal statement for each category. Time-management consultants often suggest one "life goal." I believe women's lives encompass too much for that to be practical. My own greatest stress came from trying to name my top priority— until I saw I must daily juggle several "top" priorities. Now, because I live in many arenas (personal, professional, family, church, and community), I have specific goals for each. That gives direction for planning months, weeks, and days and also gives me criteria for

saying yes or no to other people's requests. Appendix A contains two sample life-goal statements.

Remember:

These are your goals. Nobody can set goals that work for you except you. Even you will revise them throughout your life. Don't write what you fear is the least you can do but what you hope is the most you can do. Picture yourself perfect and describe that! (Perfect for you, not perfect for your best friend or Superwoman.)

2. Take a second look. Back off for a minute and ask a different question: If I knew I would die in six months, what would I want to be sure to have done in each category of my life? Assume your funeral and cemetery plot are taken care of. Concentrate on how you want to *live* until then. Write it down.

3. Compare your initial life-goal statement with these new "If-I-had-only-six-months-to-live" goals. Do you want to revise your original goals? When I first did this exercise, I put as my family life goal "To prepare my children to live independently when they leave home." When I contemplated leaving them in six months, I wrote at once, "To enjoy my children"! My new statement in this category combines the two: "To enjoy our two sons and raise them to be God-conscious men who know they are loved, who are equipped to care for themselves, and who have experienced the joy of caring for others."

Note that we *can't* write goals for other people. I didn't say I was raising men who would care about God, care for themselves and others. That will be their decision. All I can do is provide home, church, and service situations that let them experience what I hope they will choose to become.

4. Take a third look. Redraft your old goals to reflect your short-term ones, then ask, If I accomplish these things and nothing else in my lifetime, will I have lived the best life I think I can? If you find something missing, add it now.

Remember two things:

You're not writing *plans* at this stage—not saying how you will accomplish what you want to do. You are writing what you hope to become—the vision you have in that area of your life. Dream BIG!

Don't omit the "quiet things" of life. Some of our highest goals and pleasures are quiet and may get overlooked as we write ambitious action goals. If you value family vacation times, personal meditation, time to smell the roses, be sure to include that in your goals, or it may not get done.

Who helps or hinders you from achieving your goals?

As we said in the last chapter, women know that our lives and achievements are interconnected with the lives and achievements of the people with whom we live and work.

1. As you look at your goals, then, which of them

    may bring you into conflict with someone else?
    Name the person(s).
2. How can you negotiate and reciprocate? What can
    you offer in exchange for help in meeting this
    goal? (One woman promised her spouse that if he
    would help her become a certified public accoun-
    tant, she would pay for his law school later.)
3. Whom will you need to confront? About what?
    Can you tell your mother you are going to
    become a doctor even if she has her heart set on
    your becoming a teacher? Are your goals worth
    explaining and even risking displeasure for?

Write a final life-goal statement

1. On a fresh sheet of paper, write down "finished"
    life-goal statements based on your dreams, your
    six-month goals revision, and an honest assess-
    ment of prior commitments that shape who you
    are. If you have married a quiet, gentle farmer,
    for instance, you are unlikely to have a career as
    a trapeze artist (although you could travel with a
    circus in the winter after crops are in). If you
    have borne children, you are unlikely to aban-
    don them in favor of a lifetime with Mother
    Theresa in Calcutta, but you could plan now to
    spend some time there after your children are
    grown. Remember that these goals reflect your
    thinking at this point in your life—they are not
    chiseled in stone. They may change from time to
    time, or categories may become more or less
    important in different seasons.
2. Keep your goals at eye level. Some women keep

their goals in a notebook or calendar and carry it everywhere. Other women put their goals in the Bible they use regularly. I keep mine where I see them daily. Wherever you put them, look at them often as a reminder of what you want to be working toward.

The next four chapters discuss how to make plans so our years, months, weeks, and days flow in the direction of our life goals. Two possible stumbling blocks merit special mention here.

First, old habits are hard to break. To reach new goals we have to stop running in old circles.

Second, some women have never been encouraged to consider their talents, interests, and skills. As a result, they don't know what they like to do or can do. I know several who have made dramatic changes. One was a teacher until she realized what she really loved was the paperwork. She is now a banker. One who worked with abusive children all day realized she was reliving her abused childhood and preferred working with adults. She is now a paralegal. One woman, a homemaker, discovered a talent for painting and at age sixty-three began a career as an artist. If you don't know what you can or want to do, find a counseling service at a local college or a Christian counselor who can provide exercises and wisdom to help you determine what your interests and abilities truly are.[3]

So you now have written goals for the rest of your life (or until you revise them). Let's now discuss how to put legs and feet on them and get them walking.

CHAPTER SEVEN

Planning the BIG *Picture*

People live not in the ideal world of books but in the real world of the unexpected, the accidental, and other people. This next chapter, therefore, is the trickiest. We are about to discuss setting concrete goals for this season of your life and for one year, knowing that circumstances may force any of us to alter plans.

You may feel this is an unnecessary process for you. If you spent time visioning life goals in the last chapter, you may feel ready right now to get on with this week and today. Let me urge you to go through one season's planning process. If it doesn't help in your life, perhaps life goals and intermittent planning make the most sense for you. I believe, however, that this process can help you move more purposefully into the future.

Let me tell you why I believe that.

The first time I set goals was in 1975. My husband—

weary of being a "patron of the arts" for a writer who spent most of her time reading other people's books, serving on boards and committees, or having lunch with friends—requested accountability. I sat down and drew up grand five-year goals describing an ever-increasing commitment to writing for income. I included hunger committees I felt God wanted me to serve on. I included faith growth. I included time with friends.

I did not include having two babies.

When our first child was born in 1977, I nearly killed myself staying on schedule. The spring before he was born, I completed a commissioned, full-length drama and a thirteen-week church-school curriculum. When he was four months old, I finished a book of hunger-education games—often typing at three o'clock in the morning while he dozed beside me in his swing. I dragged him to meetings and workshops all over the country. I was on target with my goals. I was also exhausted, irritable, and so busy being efficient that I often missed the fun of mothering. By the time he was two years old, I was more than willing to cut back my writing to three mornings a week and drop most other commitments. When the second baby came in 1980, I put my goals in a drawer and forgot them.

In 1989, cleaning out some files, I found those old goals. To my utter surprise, I discovered I had met every one of them—in fourteen years, not five, but I had met them. Even when I was not conscious of them, they were buried in my memory and charted my direction. They had not been discarded, merely postponed.

PROBLEMS WITH LONG-TERM GOALS

I've read many books that suggest that we set five-year, three-year, and one-year goals. Most of those books were written by men. I find that women have a hard time using those timelines, for several reasons.

For one thing, many women are discovering new possibilities for themselves at an astonishing rate. In five years we may not want what we think we want today. My own mother left teaching and became an artist at sixty-two. All of us know women who showed up at twenty-fifth college reunions living drastically different lives than anyone had expected. Bonnie said, "I once set five-year goals for myself, then discovered three years later that none of them were appropriate. I had narrowed my goals too much. I was trying to make decisions before I had evaluated my real priorities."

A second reason that five-year or three-year goals don't make sense for women is that, whether we like it or not, women's lives are usually bound up with the lives of others. No woman can say whether in five years she will be married, divorced, or widowed, working or staying at home, emptying her nest or refilling it, or even living in the same home—and few of us will make those decisions in glorious isolation! Bonnie spoke for most of us when she said, "A lot of my future depends on the people I live and work with." Maxine said, "I keep waiting for an empty nest, but they keep coming back!"

The unexpected and accidental often alter a woman's life situation more drastically than they alter the situation of the men in her life. Divorce statistics reveal that while most men get richer when they divorce, most women get poorer. I've already told how having two children delayed my own ability to achieve "five-year" goals. Similarly, when Gloria's mother became chronically and terminally ill, Gloria and her husband bought and moved into a larger home. Gloria put some of her personal goals on hold and devoted a great deal of time and energy that next year to either caring for or finding care for her mother.

A third reason that five-year and three-year goals don't make much sense for women is that women's lives, as we have said before, tend to be lived not in five-year segments, but in seasons. Those seasons have borders like "when the children go to school," "when they go to college," "as long as mother lives with me," "until retirement," "while I live in this place," or "until I finish serving on this committee." No woman can realistically set long-term goals, then, unless they relate to a current season of her life and help her prepare for what she believes will be her next season.

WHY DO WE SET LONG-TERM GOALS?

Even though long-term planning involves some pitfalls, it offers many advantages and can help reduce stress in our lives.

A WISE WOMAN KNOWS:
*"If you fail to plan,
you plan to fail."*

First, long-term planning that can move us toward our life goals *keeps us from spending our energy and time on other people's goals for our time.* Years pass, and we discover that we are no closer to our goals than when we set them!

Second, long-term planning also *helps us choose wisely between possibilities.* "Our challenges stem not from scarcity but from surplus, not from oppression but from options."[1] While this statement may not be true for all women in our society, most of us have more options than we may realize. Taking time to look several years down the road can stretch our idea of what may be possible for us.

Third, setting long-term goals both *focuses our attention on goals appropriate to our particular seasons and prevents us from letting other goals drop through the cracks of our busy days.*

Ann said, "I didn't look realistically at all of who I really am when I was setting my goals. When my girls were little and both developed juvenile diabetes, caring for them was very time consuming. I decided that I would do no more than be a good wife, mother, and teacher until they were grown. For ten years I made no effort to do more at my job than to teach five classes well. Then one day I saw a computer printout listing faculty members and years since their last promotion. I was on the top of that list!

"Years of forgotten achievement pushed to the surface. How could I have been high school salutatorian, Phi Beta Kappa in college, Harvard summer-school scholarship recipient, and Woodrow Wilson Fellow—and now be the faculty member with fewest promotions? It hurt! When setting my goals, I had failed to realize how important academic achievement really was for me. I thought I could put it all behind me and not miss it. I was wrong.

"I wish I could say to women everywhere: The Lord hasn't taken you out of the world. God has come to live with you in the world. You and God together need to look at *your* personality, *your* childhood, *your* priorities, *your* past choices, and *your* hopes in order to see what is driving you and where God wants to help you make changes and adjustments. Don't kid yourself that the things that influence and impact the rest of the world—sickness, loss of a job, pride in certain achievements—won't touch you. Of course they will. But you have resources beyond yourself to deal with those things. Plan to tap deeply and regularly into your resources of faith."

SETTING A SEASON'S GOALS

For women, I believe that setting long-term goals involves three steps:

1. Define your current season and anticipate the next one. What is the next major boundary in your life? Are there important minor boundaries between now and then? What do you expect your next season to be like?

For example, my own season while writing this book: mother of two school-age boys. Major boundaries: when each son goes to college. Important minor boundaries: when each son gets a driver's license. Each of those boundaries will mean both real losses and real freedom for me. Next season: increased work and less money while two boys attend college. Once they are out of college, I hope to have money to travel and more time to work on hunger issues. My seasonal goals deal with the time while they are still at home *and* with making plans for a life after they are gone.

    2. Prayerfully consider your life goals to see how they relate to your current and next probable season. What will you want to emphasize just now? What may you decide to put on hold or give less attention to? What will you need to do now to prepare for the next season?

Again illustrating from my own life, I realize that these years are crucial for teaching the boys what they need to know to live on their own. They are also important years to enjoy them before they leave home. Other goals can be postponed while I concentrate on family time. (If I were practicing what I preach, would I be working on this chapter while my nine-year-old makes macaroni downstairs? Yes, because I know that in these years I also must focus on writing for income to help pay their college tuitions!)

    3. Set some seasonal goals for each of your life goal categories. Also set some goals to prepare for your next season.

In my own case, I am setting goals of training the boys, being intentional about vacation and recreation times, and giving them the spiritual support they need through adolescence. I am also concentrating on writing and marketing books, and giving less time to volunteer activities than I have in past seasons. At the same time, while I must postpone travel for a few years and curtail hunger activities, I will try to keep informed about issues and am already beginning to look for opportunities I can take advantage of later.

One span I do *not* like to see women plan for is "until I get married." When a woman puts off planning what to do or become because she hopes to find somebody to help shape that, one of two things is likely to happen: she doesn't get married, and as a result she remains "shapeless" for too many years; or she marries somebody who can help shape her and discovers she doesn't like the shape! In marriage, two become one. But I believe (and see) that marriages are healthier when each of the two knows who he or she is and doesn't expect to reflect the other. Marriage is for people, not mirrors.

A WORD ABOUT ANNUAL GOALS

Even if you prefer not to set long-term goals, do set measurable, attainable one-year goals. They form the base on which to plan your months, weeks, and days.

Eventually you may want to set them just before your birthday or between Christmas and New Year's Day, evaluating how well you have met last year's goals before setting those for a new year. Begin by setting them now. You can always revise them later.

EXERCISE

Find pencil, paper, and your life goals from the last chapter.

What are your goals for this season?

1. Decide what your next logical boundary is (preferably, but not necessarily, less than ten years away). At the top of your paper write: Seasonal Goals to Be Reached by [the date for accomplishing these goals].
2. Look at your life-goal statement. For each category, ask yourself, What could I do in this next season of life to begin to achieve this goal? List every idea you have, no matter how silly.
3. Consider your lists and prayerfully make a realistic estimate of what you really might achieve in this time. (You may find that one of your silliest ideas combines with one of your others for a great annual goal.)

For instance, if you share my goal of seeing much of the world in your lifetime, perhaps seeing one country is realistic in the next eight years. Or perhaps you can't afford to visit the countries at this point in your life, but you can learn more about the countries you want to see—learn a language, read library books about the countries, or invite a foreign college student or business person to your home for a holiday. Or maybe you could check out a public television news item about courier services that let you fly very cheaply to various countries.

Similarly, if your goal is to learn to know, love, and serve God, what will you do in the next five years to come closer to God? Begin or extend private study/prayer time? Read a specified number of faith-expanding books? Join or start a small prayer group?

Teach children's church school so you are forced to learn the Bible better?

Note: Make *measurable* goals! Even if they are to point a direction, you need to know as clearly as possible what direction they are pointing.

4. Write a one-sentence, seasonal goal statement for each of your life goals. See Appendix A for samples.
5. Consider all your goals from a financial angle. Will any require more money than you now have? If so, what steps will you take to begin to get that money? Some ideas: save a small amount regularly; find a better-paying job; get more education to increase your salary; do some extra part-time work, cut current expenses. Chapter 13 further discusses the relationship between money and goals.

What are your one-year goals?

1. Consider your seasonal goals for each category. What steps could you take in these next twelve months to achieve them? Write down *all* steps.
2. Here's a curve ball. Under each category, write down all the other things you are already committed to in each area, with specific time allocations: teaching Sunday school 50 Sundays, chairing the Women's Circle meeting 6 times, etc.

You can't fool me. I know you have on your calendar things that aren't on your goals list! This year, at least. Eventually you may want to change that—by expanding your goals or eliminating some of what you are doing. But at this stage, your one-year list should include all the commitments you already have made as well as new ones you want to take on.

3. Cull. Obviously, if one goal is to reduce stress in our lives, it's not wise to make unattainable lists of what we want to do in this next year! Look at the one-year goals you have written and ask:

— What in ten years would I regret not having done?

— What in ten years would I probably not remember doing?

— What could I do better if I waited for another life season?

— What do I need more of in my life?

—What do I need less of in my life?

Cut your list to two to four items in each category—fewer if your list seems too long. (Remember that no matter how well you made your list, you still have to cook and eat a certain number of meals, do a certain amount of laundry, bake cookies for a number of unexpected events, and entertain unexpected guests this year.)

4. Keep all these lists at eye level. Review your annual goals monthly, the others at least annually and revise as necessary.

Now you have a life plan. Let's get on with making it work!

CHAPTER EIGHT

You Gotta Be You!

I once had a roommate who spent an hour and a half getting ready for work. She would wash her face, then sit on her bed and think a bit. She would brush her hair, slowly, and sit on her bed some more. When she cooked a meal, she drifted around the kitchen for two hours or more. When she started a sentence, you sat back and waited.

Now I have a son just like her. His path from the house to the car can take him all over the lot. Gathering clothes from his floor for the laundry can take most of an afternoon, for he builds a block Alamo en route. When he washes dishes, he dreams over the bubbles. When he takes a shower, he squats down in the tub and organizes an entire Star Wars battle—absolutely forgetting that he was on his way to bed.

Since I tend to move quickly, talk quickly, and work best under pressure, we sometimes drive each other crazy. We're like Santa's reindeer—a Dasher and a Dancer!

People are different in other ways too. Some people see clutter as signs of disorganization. For others, clutter means a major creative project going on. Organization for them may show up in tidy drawers and well-kept files or in a constant flow of creativity that rises from seeming chaos. If you aren't sure which a woman is, read her refrigerator magnets!

I'm still working on accepting that *different* is not necessarily *wrong*. Several years ago my husband and I took the Myers Briggs Personality Inventory, a test that describes in detail the strengths of many personality types. It gave us labels for why Bob gets totally involved in a project like painting the dining-room ceiling (he's a Sensate) and why I get frantic if he's not done when guests are due in fifteen minutes (I'm an Intuitive). We now understand why Bob argues from the vantage point of logic (he's a Thinker) while I push for values I feel are important (being a Feeler). Probably the best thing that test did for our marriage was to put both styles of living on a chart of Acceptable Behaviors. We don't always live on the mountaintop of acceptance, but we climb it now and then.

When I started this book, I was tempted to write only to sisters like me—dashers who prefer exterior clutter and interior organization—and let other women write books for their own kind. But as I interviewed effective, grace-filled women who have overcome enormous amounts of stress in their lives, I realized they are all different. To learn from their wisdom, we must also look at their various styles.

As you consider how this book can best help you organize your own unique life, take into frequent account the kind of person you are. Do you thrive on pressure, or do you hate it? Do you prefer an organized life, or do you prefer to "go with the flow" except when you suffer from overflow? When company is coming and you start to clean house, is it because you like things to look nice or because you worry what they will say about you or because you want them to have at least one chair to sit on? I know all of those women—and women who are like none of them.

A friend, hearing I was writing this book, sent me Anne Ortlund's *Disciplines of a Beautiful Woman*. Anne organizes her life by keeping everything she needs—goals, notebook, to-do lists, calendar, Bible study notes and journal—in one notebook that she carries everywhere.

I found many helpful tips in her book, but her notebook wouldn't work for me. If I organized my life in one notebook, I would lose the notebook! I need things filed, pegged onto my bulletin board, or sorted in various baskets (more on baskets in chapter 11). I don't even mind occasionally scrabbling through piles, if I know what's in the pile. And some days I'm downright disorganized. On one of those days I received a note from school saying, "Your son lost his homework. Please sign and return this note." I had to send another note. "Sorry, I've lost your note. It runs in the family." Each of us has to create systems that work for us.

Elise is highly organized. We talked while she was getting her nails sculptured—the only "sit-down" hour she expected to have that week. She said, "I'm super organized. Nobody I know lives her life like I do. I'm a partner in a law firm and have three offices scattered in two cities. Most of my clients, however, are elderly people who need me to go to them, so I practically live in my car—I dictate in the car, talk on the phone in the car, even change clothes in the car when I have to. I carry with me anything that I could possibly need—all my jewelry, my cosmetics, essential office supplies.

"I also keep our house very organized. That's important to me. What is not essential for me to do, I hire done. I spend the first hour of every day planning what the housekeeper should do, looking at my calendar for the day, and calling my mother, who does all my shopping. Her help over the last twenty-five years of child rearing and professional life has been pivotal. Without her it would never have been as much fun—or as possible, although I had a home office when the children were very small and later scheduled appointments so I would be home when they came home from school. My youngest daughter will go to college this fall.

"I couldn't live without my calendar. It contains every single thing I need to know about today, this week, and this month, and all the telephone numbers I need both professionally and socially. I'm constantly looking for ways to use time better."

Maxine and I met on a lazy Sunday afternoon in her living room, while her husband entertained my husband with pictures from their recent trip to Alaska. She said, "I have an ordered life, but not a disciplined life. I don't plan much what I'll be doing in five years—one job just seems to follow another. I do concentrate on four areas—education, the humane society, health, and missions. I don't take responsibilities in any other area.

"I work half time just now as a medical technologist. I like mornings, so I have arranged to start work at half-past four. I get up at three o'clock A.M., jog, work eight hours, then take an afternoon nap. I still have a good bit of the day left for meetings and things. At one time I tried teaching nursing lab courses. Talk about stress! I'm not a teacher, and I didn't like it at all. That taught me to concentrate on what I do best.

"Our children are all through college now except the oldest, who has gone back for a graduate degree. When they were little, sometimes I would get real organized at home. We would have chore lists and schedules. But that usually went out the window. I didn't even insist that they clean their rooms. Their rooms are their rooms. When they were small, I cleaned their rooms real well and told them I wouldn't come back to clean until they were each eighteen. I'm not much on housework anyway. My husband tells me there *are* women who dust between July 4 and Christmas. I'm not one of them, unless there's something special going on."

Of course, "something special" at Maxine's can be a sit-down dinner for forty, a wedding reception in her gorgeous yard, a school-board brunch, or a birthday party for a ninety-seven-year-old friend. Perhaps one reason Maxine doesn't have to clean "regularly" is that she entertains so often. That works for her.

Gail and I met for lunch two weeks before her

younger daughter's wedding. Gail has worked outside the home for only two brief periods, but she has been an almost full-time volunteer in church and community organizations for many years. Among ministries she has helped start in her city are a shelter for pre-delinquent teens, a CROP walk for hunger, a Food Bank annual fund-raising banquet, and a program to sponsor refugees. She currently also teaches fifth-grade Sunday school, teaches a twice-monthly Bible class for migrant children, and serves on numerous local church and presbytery committees.

"I'm fortunate my husband's a judge," she said. "He has always worked such regular hours that he could be home in the evening with the children when they were little, freeing me to go to meetings. He helped them with homework and did many of the dishes." She chuckled. "I'd come home and say, 'Who did the dishes?' and he'd say, 'The parakeet.' Housework usually has come second with me. Luckily we had a new house that didn't need much cleaning. My schedule was so irregular I never had special days to clean or do laundry. The chores just got done when we needed them.

"I'm involved in many things, but it seems I've most enjoyed starting new areas of mission. I get inspired by a need, start a project, and turn it over to other people."

Bonnie and I ate lunch together at her home, which is also her office. We talked between incoming calls and one visitor. She said, "I used to resist a disciplined life because it felt so rigid. I'm a people person. I wanted to get tasks done so I could be with people. I thought a disciplined, ordered life meant I couldn't take time for people. I'm learning what *my* order is.

"I'm a night person, so I have my quiet time at night when nobody is around. I also do office work late—often until two o'clock in the morning. I'm seldom (never, by preference) at my desk before ten o'clock, and I schedule people into my days—lunches like this, one day a week at a hospital as a chaplain's assistant.

"I've discarded some disciplines I had imposed on myself, for I see now that they were others' rules for my life. For a while, on someone else's recommendation, I spent half an hour every morning in meditative prayer. I learned that not only do I not pray clearly in the morning (I don't even think clearly in the morning), but that's not a natural way for me to pray. Instead, I have a running conversation with God all day, and I meditate when I'm working with plants or cutting vegetables for lunch. To sit down and say 'Now I am going to meditate' is foreign to who I am."

YOU GOTTA HAVE RHYTHM!

As these women illustrate, part of our uniqueness is a personal chemical rhythm. We can let it work for us or against us. The trick is to decide what, for you, is the prime time of day. Are you a morning person, ready to face the world and take on big challenges before eight o'clock in the morning? Or do you prefer late-night quiet? (One way for married people to answer that question is look at your spouse—you often are whatever he is not!) How much sleep does your body need? When are you most likely to get drowsy or have the least energy?

Our days also have a rhythm structured by the schedules of others—when children are in school, when work begins, when groups meet. Looking at our day's rhythm, then, also involves looking at when we get large blocks of uninterrupted time and when our time is, at best, piecemeal.

Answers to those questions can help us schedule big, creative, or just plain hard tasks for prime, uninterrupted time and can help us save low-energy times (downtime) or piecemeal time for piddles and putters—calling the dentist, writing bills, getting a haircut, folding laundry, doing routine office tasks.

A WISE WOMAN KNOWS:
*"If you spend minutes wisely,
hours and days take care of themselves."*

One time-management expert recommends using the early morning for phone calls and minor tasks, late morning for creative and big tasks, after lunch for minor tasks while lunch digests, and late afternoon to plan your next day. Obviously he doesn't plan his schedule around precious hours when children are in preschool, late afternoon pandemonium when everybody is suddenly home at once, or midnight laundry after a long day at his office. Also, he obviously has no friends like Bonnie who strenuously object to being called before ten o'clock in the morning. But on his skeleton of a typical day—early morning, late morning, early afternoon, late afternoon, and, for women, evening—we can add the meat of those things we want and have to do.

In addition to understanding our daily rhythms, we also need to look at our weekly, monthly, and annual rhythms—scheduled events or seasons that cause predictable pressure. Merchants, ministers, and room mothers, for instance, know that Christmas will be a hectic, exhausting time. Parents and educators know that the beginning and end of the school year will be rough. If you've ever toilet trained a child in a day (or over several weeks), you know that's not the best season to toss in a sit-down dinner for twenty. Bureaucrats and leaders in organizations know that around the time of annual meetings and publication deadlines, tempers wear thin.

What surprises me is how seldom we take that into account when planning annual schedules for our homes and workplaces. Taking time to plot an annual "stress" calendar—noting when the peak stress will occur, blocking out time ahead of it to prepare and downtime afterwards for family or co-workers—can increase both morale and productivity. I heartily recommend "recuperation time" as a valid schedule entry both for office and home calendars!

Betty said, "At the Community of Celebration in Aliquippa, we work very hard to meet publishing and recording deadlines. Then we take an evening and go out for an elegant meal, or we rent a movie and make popcorn. We are, after all, the Community of *Celebration*. Taking time to celebrate our achievements—and recover from them—is very important to us."

Other more subtle rhythms also contribute to

stress. I once worked in an office that scheduled our regular staff meeting for the same Tuesday each month. Three of four women staff members were on identical birth-control-pill cycles and started their periods on that very day each month. One day in despair our boss asked, "What's the matter with the women in this office? Get you into a staff meeting and you turn into grouches." We told him why. Moving that staff meeting to another day of the month did a good bit to improve working relationships.

Obviously, not all workplaces or family schedules will be set by women's menstrual cycles. And we wouldn't advocate that. I do believe, however, that a concept of rhythm is something women can offer working environments.

I once worked simultaneously for two large church boards, half time in each. One was a staff of all women, the other was an executive staff dominated by men (hereafter called "the men"). The two staffs had very different work styles. The women had two casual prayer and sharing times a week, with dough-nuts and coffee. The men had a prepared devotional by one of the ministers each Friday, but staff members were often too busy to attend. The women took a daily coffee break where executives and clerical staff all caught up on each other's lives. The men drank coffee at their desks. The women met once a month for a potluck lunch to hear about conferences and staff travels and to celebrate joys like the birth of a great-niece. The men met once a week for a bag-lunch staff meeting. The women had a monthly birthday party. The men never had a party except for evening (after-hours) dinners. The women expected staff members who traveled to take "comp" time when they had been on the road overnight and on weekends. The men expected staff members who traveled to be back on time the next day. Both groups accomplished enormous amounts of work. One group also had fun and made lifetime friends.

Of course, we all know women who buy into the "men's" type of office management and men who prefer the "women's" style. A friend of mine divides people into two types: workers and players. I don't think it's that simple. I believe that all workers can find ways to play, and players accomplish a lot of work. The important thing is to get in touch with the rhythms within and without us and to make certain we provide balanced time for "all things under heaven," not just for work.

EXERCISE

Find your prime, uninterrupted time

1. Discover your daily rhythm. Think about the last three days. When did you feel most energy? When were you the most drained?
2. Look at your calendar for next month in terms of early morning, late morning, early afternoon, late afternoon, evening.
3. Which blocks are best for you to use to meet important goals (times when you are at your best and have the most uninterrupted time)?
4. Which are best for you to do maintenance chores: dishes, laundry, routine work?
5. When is the best time for doing the tasks that

have no meaning in your life? (All of us spend some of our time—one writer estimates about ten percent—on that type of activity.)

6. For now, before getting down to specific planning in the next chapter, lightly shade with pencil those times in the next month when you will work on your most important goals. Pencil in times you know you can do small or piddly items. Pencil in at least one time to have fun!

Consider your upcoming annual rhythm

1. Look at the next twelve months. What do you already know is going to put you under pressure? On your calendar, block out time ahead of each to "prepare for pressure." If you thrive on deadlines, your time may be immediately before the deadline; carefully guard that time. If you prefer to work a bit at a time, plan to start soon enough to avoid the pressure you hate. If you know some of the steps you will have to take— buy school clothes, write an annual report— pencil them in too. Promise yourself that if others want to intrude on that time, you will resist strongly!

2. Block out time after pressure times to "recuperate." Dream about one or two celebrations you would enjoy.

Now, finally, we are ready to talk about prayerfully taking charge of life so that we have time to do what is most important for each of us—and to do it with a modicum of grace and joy. Like driving and reading, managing our time is a learned skill. We can all do it!

Let us now consider when to plan, how to plan, and the actual mechanics of planning a year, a month, and a week.

CHAPTER NINE

The Time Is Now

When is the best time to plan? The answer to that is, what time do you have?

Annual planning can take an hour or more. I usually do mine the week before a new year begins. Monthly and weekly planning take less time. I like Sunday afternoons or evenings. Some women choose the night their spouse goes bowling, Monday mornings after the children leave for school, or one lunch hour at the office. Some people say you should always plan early in the morning or at the end of a day. I say, find your own best time—whenever you can block out prime, uninterrupted time.

HOW DO WE PLAN?

Once we decide what we want to do (our annual goals), planning involves four steps:

1. breaking goals into time-sequenced tasks,
2. bracketing tasks into components,
3. looking for related tasks, and
4. deciding when we will do each task.

A WISE WOMAN KNOWS:
*"You don't do goals;
you do tasks to meet goals."*

Tasks come in three sizes:

Big tasks take more than thirty minutes: papering a bedroom, planning vacation church school, writing an annual report, or completing this chapter.

Small tasks take from ten minutes to half an hour: picking up the wallpaper and papering supplies, calling people to bring cookies to vacation church school, or writing a memo to others who have to help with the annual report. (There are no small tasks involved in writing this chapter!)

Instant tasks take less than ten minutes: calling the wallpaper store to check on hours, picking up cookies for vacation church school while you are in the grocery store, or finding last year's annual report (if you know where it is).

Tasks also come in two weights: critical and not so critical. Critical tasks can be any size—as big as furnishing a house or office, as small as calling your sister on her birthday.

The issue, as we plan, is when to schedule tasks

that require big chunks of time, how to make sure that small critical tasks get priority, and how to fit in little or less critical tasks so they don't consume our lives.

We follow a planning process whenever we fix a meal. Consider a menu of fried chicken, rice and gravy, green beans southern style (cooked an hour or more), Jello, and iced tea. We don't fry the chicken and set it aside while we put on water for the rice, then, when the rice is done, begin to string beans or make the Jello—at least, most of us don't.

Most of us automatically

- make a shorthand mental list of what tasks have to be done in what order for each menu item ("fry chicken" really means cut up chicken, wash it, heat oil, batter meat, fry forty minutes);
- group some items into components that can be completed ahead and set aside (wash, string, and snap the beans);
- identify related tasks (boil water for both tea and Jello);
- plan exactly when we will do what (make Jello hours ahead, fry chicken and cook beans an hour ahead, get ice and make the gravy when we are almost ready to sit down).

As we proceed through our checklist— *voila!* —a whole meal is completed!

Planning also involves keeping our pulse on the flow of our lives. Betty said, "Two things make me frantic, and they sound like a paradox. One is when my life gets too 'bitty,' when I have too many irons in the fire and I'm moving all over the place doing a bit of this and a bit of that. The other is if I get so carried away in one area of my life that I let everything else slide. One day when I was writing a song, my daughter asked me to do something for her. I put it off, reluctant to stop. She asked again and again, and I kept putting her off. Finally she stormed in and said, 'Mama, you forgot and got and got!' We need to find a balance."

A WISE WOMAN KNOWS:
*"The point of planning
is to decrease stress.
Don't settle for anything less."*

In the following pages I explain a detailed planning process. Before we get into the process, let me speak a word of warning: While a certain amount of planning is necessary and helpful, too much planning can be harmful and can keep us from doing other things. Experiment until you discover how much planning you need to do to manage stress in your own life.

KEEPING OUR FAMILIES OFF THE ALTAR

Many businesses now require employees to set annual work goals. I have found by painful experience that unless we mesh work goals with personal, family, and service goals, one sabotages the other. When work goals take priority over family, the family suffers; when both adults work at jobs that take priority, the suffering is acute. It can even be fatal to the family unit.

My husband concludes that people put work goals first because they have never taken time to set personal or family goals. Perhaps. I believe people give priority to their work goals because some of them genuinely believe their professional goals are more important than their personal goals or even their families. Those whose jobs are seen as ministry or service, especially, are likely to see putting their jobs first as "presenting our bodies [and our families] as a living sacrifice to God" through the "good" we do. We need to remember that Jesus set an example of regular withdrawal from his work for both solitude and intimate time with disciples.

Donna provides another insight about why we value professional goals more highly than personal goals. "When I update my resume, I can measure how I'm progressing toward meeting professional goals. Family and personal goals are harder to evaluate. I find almost no way to measure family goals until the children are grown or until we can look back after many years of marriage. The logbook of family and personal goals is our lives."

No matter how difficult it is at first, women must learn to balance personal, family, and professional goals, giving each its proper weight, to insure that we give as much attention to who we are becoming as we give to what we are doing.

PLANNING A YEAR

Planning to meet annual goals requires uninterrupted time, a quiet place, paper, pencil, and a calendar with enough space to write in everything you want to remember. Then you won't have to be organized—your calendar will be, instead.

Whether you have both an office calendar and a home calendar or just one that contains everything depends largely on how much your office impinges on your home. If your job is regular, seldom if ever encroaching on your home schedule, then you can keep a calendar at work and one at home. On the other hand, if your work involves shifts, emergency calls, evening or weekend meetings, or out-of-town trips, you'd better keep home and work calendars together! In either case, on a monthly and weekly basis, mesh calendars for all family members to avoid double scheduling and time conflicts.

EXERCISE

Appendix A illustrates the complete planning process, from personal life-goal statements through annual, monthly, weekly, and daily plans.

1. List all big tasks needed to meet each of your annual goals. (We'll consider small or instant tasks later.)
2. Put tasks in time sequence. Number tasks in order, showing which tasks must or can be done first before others.
3. Look for component parts. If two or more tasks on a list can be done together, then pick a time when you can do them all.
4. Look for related tasks or tasks that could accomplish more than one goal. Mark them with a personal code.

5. Establish a schedule.
6. Beside each task, write the month or months in which you plan to do it. (Meeting the goal of learning a new habit means steady, regular—often daily—work.)
7. Make lists of monthly tasks for all your goals. You will use these lists in monthly planning.
8. As you consider the year ahead and the amount of work needed to accomplish some goals, you may decide they are multi-year goals. Divide your tasks accordingly. Which tasks will you do this year? Which next?

PLANNING A MONTH

Once you know exactly what steps you need to take to accomplish your annual goals and which should be done in which months, planning a month ahead is a matter of looking at work and home calendars and meshing what you have already scheduled with time to work toward annual goals.

A WISE WOMAN KNOWS:
"Never sacrifice the important on the altar of the urgent."

EXERCISE

Make sure you have *all* family work and home calendars available. Pressure in one place *always* impinges on the other. You also need this month's task list(s).

Write what you already know

1. On your home calendar, pencil in every scheduled item—sports practices, luncheon dates, Bible studies, once-a-week volunteer jobs, out-of-town trips for any household member, school or work holidays, PTA meetings, guests, and anything else you need to remember. Anything you leave out can sabotage you later. For your office calendar (or on the same one, if you combine them) write in every scheduled trip, meeting, deadline, or appointment.

2. Compare calendars for major deadlines. Mark all stress times on both calendars (for instance, draw a yellow line through days of pressure at home or at work) so you can know at once to ease up on other commitments.

3. If you live with other people, compare monthly calendars. Note conflicts and schedules that affect one another. (Will you have to drive a carpool? Will you need to bring refreshments to the meeting? Will your spouse or roommate or close friend be out of town that week, leaving you to cope alone?) Also note each person's pressure days so the family can provide additional support. For major times of stress, plan ahead for easier meals, some kind of recreation, and a letdown period afterward.

4. Consider upcoming special events like birthdays and anniversaries. Pencil in on the appropriate date anything you must do ahead to get ready. For example, if your mother's birthday is

the 18th, when must you buy the gift? When should you get it in the mail?

5. Are you comfortable with the month's flow at this point? (We all know calendars don't really fill up until a week ahead.) Do you have blocks of time to work on important goals, complete big projects, and meet deadlines? If you don't see any time to work on a goal you want to work on, what can you combine or eliminate at this point? Can you start a carpool for the new soccer season? Could a conference call replace an out-of-town trip?

6. Look for this month's (and next month's) deadlines that aren't a part of meeting your important goals. Break each task into smaller ones and pencil in when you will need to do each part to be ready on time and avoid undue pressure.

Put on the calendar monthly tasks that will lead to annual goals

1. Compare your calendar and your list of this month's big tasks that will move you toward your goals. Do most of this month's big tasks already appear on the calendar? If not, what blocks of time can you use for big or critical tasks? Claim them—so nobody else does. We'll worry about smaller tasks when we talk about weeks.

It takes about thirty days to establish a habit. If you are trying to establish a new one (prayer time, going to bed earlier), write it in daily for one month. When you get into a routine that includes the habit as part of your regular schedule, you can skip that. For now, it's better to err by writing too much rather than too little.

2. At the end of each month, look at the tasks that didn't get done. What do you want to do with those—drop them? delay them? add them to the next month's list?

A word of caution: Sometimes we don't do a task because we are truly procrastinating (chapter 12 explores the pitfalls of procrastinating). But sometimes we don't do a task because it's no longer appropriate or it's not really as high a priority as we thought it would be. Don't be afraid to evaluate and toss tasks when you need to. This is *your* task list—you are not being graded on how well you complete it!

3. What will you do for fun this month? Put that on the calendar too.

PLANNING A WEEK

John W. Lee, whose time-management video "Speaking of Success" I found in the public library, estimates that for every minute we spend planning our week, we save between five and fifteen minutes later. Thirty minutes of planning, then, can save over seven hours a week. (More than thirty minutes spent planning a week, he believes, becomes less effective.) Planning a week is very much like planning a month, but the process is shorter and more precise.

By this time, your calendar(s) will have gotten fuller. You will be making a costume for Thursday's skit (if you are lucky and get that much advance notice); you suddenly will have to fly across the country to solve a business crisis; the boss will have remembered the annual report was due yesterday; or you will have gotten a call reminding you that you promised six months ago to teach church school starting next Sunday. You will have added all those items to this week's calendar, of course, as they came along.

Now you are ready to consider this hectic upcoming week and decide how to get some time for what you really want to do.

EXERCISE

1. Update your week's calendar. Check with other family members or co-workers to coordinate your weeks. Also look back at the past week to pick up items that still need to be done.
2. Put legs under your life goals. If you've been doing these exercises, you've already blocked out time this week to work on tasks toward your long-term and life goals. Break each activity down into specific tasks of appropriate sizes. Small tasks can be accomplished in breaks between other activities; instant tasks use tiny chunks of time—to make a phone call or pick up something en route to somewhere else. Tasks of various sizes also offer more chances for you to feel the satisfaction of accomplishing your goals.

A WISE WOMAN KNOWS:
*"Never underestimate
the power of pride in
one task well done."*

129

3. Look ahead to upcoming weeks. If you hate working under pressure, you will be working each week this month toward next month's D-day. What steps do you need to take this week to move you toward a panic-free deadline? If you thrive on pressure, what deadlines are now close enough for you to start working to meet them? When in the week will you work toward your deadlines? Claim that time too.

4. Look at the flow of your week. Will it be too much of just one thing? What breaks can you plan? Does it look all chopped into bits and pieces by too many different commitments? What can be eliminated or postponed?

5. What are you going to do for fun this week? When are you going to do it? You may think I'm a fun fanatic. Actually Bob and I are both workaholics. It wasn't until he was out of work for nearly a year that we discovered the importance of small doses of recreation. Someone asked me, "How can you all laugh so much in this situation?" We laughed because we took time to enjoy life and each other in small, inexpensive ways: a family bike ride, an evening at a local pool or beach, renting a movie and making popcorn and lemonade, playing a family game, sitting down to three games of solitaire, reading a book for sheer pleasure. It took unemployment to teach us the wisdom of balance in all parts of our lives.

A word about evaluation

Evaluation is such a dry word, I think. Gloria brought
it to life when she said, "I review my life goals every
year between Christmas and New Year's Day as well
as in September when Herb and I spend a week at the
beach. I ask, 'What is my life saying to me now? What
is God saying to me through this review? Where is
God leading me in this coming year? What direction
is God setting for me?' At the end of the year I celebrate reaching goals and see what I want to do in the
coming year. My goals deal more with my profession
and my call to ministry than with my family relationships. Perhaps I need to grow toward expanding
those goals too."

Beth said, "Periodically I evaluate my goals. Am I
heavy on one side? Spending too little time somewhere else? I also know it's easy for my children, especially the younger ones, to get lost in the shuffle, so I
have to ask how much time I'm spending with them."

I evaluate each month as well as each year, just to
see which tasks were achieved, whether those
achievements have moved me closer to where I want
to be at the end of the year, what tasks didn't get
done, and why (Did I put them off? Did I overesti-
mate what I could accomplish? Are these tasks of real
value to me?). Annually, I review to see if what I've
done in the past year has moved me closer to where I
want to be at the end of the current season.

Planning, as we have said before, is the tool we use
to shape our lives into what we think we want them
to be and do. Evaluation, or review, sharpens the tool.

CHAPTER TEN

Getting a Handle on Today

Where does the time go? We all have twenty-four hours a day, seven days a week, twelve months a year. Why do some women seem able to accomplish so much, while others get so little done?

While writing this book, I met Martha, who expressed a high level of frustration with her current schedule. "For twenty-five years we were missionaries in Korea. I raised four children and taught missionary children. I taught English classes at two universities, two seminaries, and a factory, and served as advisor for an English-language student newspaper. I wrote three hours a day. Each month we averaged 135 guest meals and nine overnight guests. Yet I was never as stressed as I am now that we are back in the States. In Korea I seemed to have so much more time and money and did things that seemed of more value to the kingdom of God. Why?"

As Martha considered her own question, she found

several answers. In Korea she hired a cook and house-keeper. Now she spends an average of five hours a day cooking, doing dishes, and cleaning. In Korea she lived near where she worked; now she drives one hour each way. "That's seven hours out of each day," she realized. "No wonder I'm so stressed out!"

She is also frustrated with the U.S. church. "So much that we do seems self-serving, self-feeding. So little time is spent preaching good news to the poor, healing the sick, setting free the oppressed—what Jesus came to do and calls us to do. Living as Jesus did is hard. The church should make it easier. Instead, it often makes it harder by robbing time and energy we need for ministry."

FINDING MORE MINUTES IN A DAY

Have you ever calculated how much time you spend in a year on traveling to and from work, sitting in meaningless meetings, or performing routine chores?

Consider the time you spend making beds. If you pull up sheets, blankets, and spread, adjust a dust ruffle, shove pillows into shams and arrange them, it takes about five minutes a day. Not much? In a year, that's thirty hours and twenty-five minutes—nearly four eight-hour working days! Considering all we do, no wonder we are overwhelmed.

A WISE WOMAN KNOWS:
*"What I can do is
what I can do,
and what I can do is enough."*

Altering habits reduces time spent on dreary tasks and frees time for what we really want to do with our lives. I don't want to suggest that we shouldn't go to work, sit through meetings, or make beds again (although my children would vote for that). I do urge you to calculate time spent on routine matters of low value to you and decide whether you could do them faster, less often, or not at all.

Making intentional decisions about how to spend our time gives us power over our days. Reducing time spent in routine chores also give us minutes and ultimately hours to accomplish more important tasks at a leisured, enjoyable pace.

In his excellent book *Ordering Your Private World*, Gordon MacDonald discusses what he calls "unseized time"—time over which we haven't taken authority. He argues convincingly that unless we take steps to order our own lives, our "unseized time" will flow naturally in four directions:

— toward those things we do least well, and which therefore take the most time to do;

— toward the demands of dominant people in our life;

— toward crises and emergencies;

— and toward what gives us the most public acclaim.[1]

A WISE WOMAN KNOWS:
*"When Jesus gave his disciples
authority over all things,
that included their time."*

What gets neglected are those quiet, important things we have always wanted to do and somehow never find the time for. They are the ones least likely to clamor for attention, least likely to cause crises or emergencies, least likely to matter to others.

Finding time for the quiet, important things takes a measure of discipline. "To bring organization to the private world where Christ chooses to live is both a lifelong and a daily matter," MacDonald has discovered. "Something within—the Bible calls it sin— resists both His residence and all of the resulting order."[2]

Taking authority over our days involves thinking through what we do. Our goal should not be to become hyperorganized, highly efficient super-women; our goal should be to spend most of our time on what we value most. To paraphrase St. Paul: Though we make many lists and never waste a minute, if we fail to achieve what we value, we have achieved nothing. Now abide these three: planning, efficiency, and effectiveness. The greatest of these is effectiveness.

TO DO OR NOT TO DO

A to-do list is nothing more than jottings of all those things we don't want to have to carry around in our brains all day—appointments, errands we need to run, calls we need to make, people we need to see, groceries we need to buy, bills we need to pay—nothing exciting, nothing even particularly interesting much of the time. Ah, but a good to-do list can be one of a woman's most powerful organizing tools.

Who should make a to-do list? Some time-management experts say unequivocally, "Anybody who wants to succeed in life." But Betty has discovered that in her own life, "I have to be careful not to make too many lists. I was such a structure maniac and a list person that one of the first things the Holy Spirit said to me was, 'Put down your lists.' I was so addicted to being in control of my day that I was not free to hear the Spirit. Now I make lists to remind me of what needs to be done, but they are always tentative. If the Spirit needs me elsewhere, that's where I go."

With that warning in mind, what goes on a to-do list? Consultants disagree on whether lists should be very long to spur us on to higher aspirations tomorrow or whether they should be limited to what is physically possible today. My own opinion is that to-do lists should be made prayerfully and include anything you don't want to forget.

I personally never put on a to-do list things that already appear on my calendar, for since I consult both daily, that wastes time. I never put on big items, like "write chapter 10," for that's what I plan to spend most of today doing. I do list "return movies to library," for that's something I could easily forget while struggling with chapter 10.

If checking off tasks gives you great satisfaction, however (and when you first start making to-do lists, it should), you may want to include both scheduled and unscheduled items. Otherwise, after a week of sixteen scheduled meetings you can wind up depressed at having not accomplished a single thing on your list!

I once read (and forgot where) a tip I believe in: Put on to-do lists not only urgent items but also important ones. Otherwise our lives are driven by whatever is urgent. A to-do list should give equal space to "get boys' library cards" and "call termite inspector." It should include "visit shut-in from church" as well as "pick up cleaning before going out of town."

From time to time, when making a to-do list, scan your annual- and monthly-goals lists again (you do keep them where you see them often, don't you?) and ask, What could I do today to move toward one of my goals?

A good to-do list, like many dinner menus, also includes yesterday's major leftovers. If something appears for several days in a row, however, either drop it or examine why you are procrastinating (see chapter 11).

Where do you keep a to-do list? Some people, especially those who prefer one notebook for everything, keep them with their calendars and carry them everywhere. Their lists include everything from surgery to grocery lists. Since I work at home, I keep my to-do list on my desk, and I keep an ongoing grocery list in the kitchen, where it gets picked up by the person leaving the house to run other errands. We seldom make a trip specifically to buy groceries.

Bonnie had a clever idea. "I used to make to-do lists every day. But when things didn't get done and I had to write them over and over, I would get angry with myself. Now my to-do tasks are written on little Post-it notes, and any that don't get done are easily transferred to the next page. Each night I organize what I want to do the next day, and if I don't get everything done, it's easy to move it on."

LEARNING THE THREE Ds

The three Ds of daily management are *drop*, *delay*, and *delegate*.

A WISE WOMAN KNOWS:
"Work smarter, not harder!"

Dropping involves looking at each item and asking, "Will it really matter if I never do this?" If the answer is no, that item can be dropped. The types of items we can drop range from eating lunch with someone out of a sense of duty to attending a weekly Bible study where we learn nothing. But dropping can be very hard.

Dropping means admitting we committed ourselves to something trivial. That may raise questions about other items, as well—what if the whole list turns out to be trivial? The answer, of course, is that we discover we have a lot more free time to get on with important things. When Francis of Assisi rejected an offer to manage his father's vast textile business, he had time to become a saint! Blessed are you when your to-do list turns up blank, for then your Heavenly Parent can fill it up.

Delaying means "Does this really have to be done today?" This question has to be asked differently by different people. If you hate pressure, prefer a regular schedule, and like to work on major tasks a bit at a time, you probably schedule small tasks and segments of major tasks far enough ahead to avoid rush at the end. For you, this question asks, "What can be delayed for a day or two without increasing my stress?" For example, if you planned to pick up arts-and-crafts supplies for Vacation Bible School today but have a doctor's appointment near the crafts store tomorrow, can you delay and save an extra trip?

If, on the other hand, you are like me and thrive on pressure, you may think you have delay down to a noble art—and even feel a bit virtuous about how well you follow Jesus' admonition not to worry about tomorrow until it almost comes. For us, "Does this really have to be done today?" means "What on this list absolutely can't be delayed any longer?" It may be fine to plan Vacation Bible School lessons the week before it happens, but student materials have to be ordered in time for them to arrive. Similarly, a Christmas skit has to be written in time for children to rehearse. A turkey has to thaw a couple of days in the refrigerator. Furthermore, if we are working on a deadline for tomorrow, we can't permit anyone else to fill up our today!

Delegating means saying, "Who else can do this job almost as well as I can?" (Obviously nobody can do it quite as well, or they would be doing it.) My husband says to tell you this is a learned skill—he learned it from me in self-defense. I'm the world's best at the old line, "While you're out, would you . . . ?"

Maxine refers to delegation as, "Inviting others to be involved in what you are doing." Isn't that clever? "A woman in our church was overwhelmed by having to take her husband to daily therapy. I felt so sorry for her, I offered to do it every day the next week. When I got home and checked my calendar, I was busy every single day! So I called five other women in the church and explained what needed doing and why I couldn't do it. They could, and did." Maxine gets away with that, I point out, because people know how much of her time is already filled with service to others.

Delegation has two drawbacks. First, we can delegate something only to somebody who thoroughly understands what must be done. We sometimes fail to delegate a task, therefore, because we think we can do it faster ourselves. That's true if we do the task only once. But what if we do it thirty times? A hundred? When we calculate training for one hour now versus doing for fifty-two hours in the next year (nine minutes a day), which is the better use of our time?

A second, more subtle drawback to delegation is that we must give up power in the process. If we are the only person who does or can do a certain thing, we control that. As we begin to get more control of our lives—and to know what is and is not important for us—we can begin to relax our power over nonessentials. I appreciated Elise's comment that she paid someone else to do "all that was not absolutely essential for me to do at home." Mothering her children was something only she could do; cooking was not.

Consider tasks you perform at home, work, church, and in volunteer organizations. Can any of those be handed on to others who may have less to do and a desire to be more involved? Does any of what you currently do legitimately fit into someone else's job description? Too many homes, offices, churches, and organizations limp along at the tyranny of the urgent because too few people do too much. Delegation costs some time and power, but it frees our lives and, ultimately, increases what can be done.

LEARNING THE A, B, C'S

Once we've mastered the three Ds, the A, B, Cs are easy. Those are for remaining items on our to-do lists—ones we have to do.

Most of us live by a myth: If I do piddly chores first, I clear the decks for the important jobs. The truth is, piddly chores, like piddly paperwork, breed behind our backs. If we don't ignore them, they will fill up our lives.

Years ago I was asked to review Alan Lakein's *How to Get Control of Your Time and Your Life.* [3] It was the first book I read on this subject, and I still think it's the best. Lakein suggests that once we get our daily to-do list made, we designate each item A (very important), B (less important), or C (not important). A items are both the urgent tasks (getting a root canal) and those we have declared important (spending half an hour in prayer). C items include tasks we do not value or can postpone almost indefinitely.

The same task can be an A or a C. Mopping the floor is usually a C for me, but if guests are coming and things are sticking to the floor, mopping becomes an immediate A.

Here is Lakein's excellent advice: *do A tasks first!* That way, if you only get A tasks done, you will have done what you deemed important. More often, the glow of accomplishing something important provides energy to tackle B tasks.

What about those poor C tasks that are used to getting all the attention? Either they become urgent and clamor their way up to the A list, or they die anonymous, unlamented deaths.

COORDINATING WITH OTHERS

Other people can wreck your day. That's not merely a bad joke; it's true. Much avoidable stress comes when we fail to coordinate our own day, week, and month with those we live or work with. Beth says, "Al and I meet daily after the kids go to school. We pray over the day and go over our calendars. I wish we had started this earlier—it would have helped tremendously. It's a good sharing time too."

THE 80/20 RULE

Time-management consultants have what they call the "80/20 rule." They claim that eighty percent of all we achieve in almost any field is achieved with twenty percent of our effort, and only twenty percent achieved with the other eighty percent of the effort. Consider these other illustrations:
— 80 percent of the tasks are done by 20 percent of the people;
— 80 percent of valuable work is done in 20 percent of the time;
— 80 percent of file usage is in 20 percent of files;
— 80 percent of wearing is of 20 percent of our clothes;
— 80 percent of dinners repeat 20 percent of recipes;

— 80 percent of sales come from 20 percent of customers;

— 80 percent of all telephone calls come from 20 percent of the callers;

— 80 percent of important conversation occurs in 20 percent of conversation;

— 80 percent of most needed housecleaning is in 20 percent of the space.

Alan Lakein says, "The 80/20 rule suggests that in a list of ten items, doing two of them will yield most (80 percent) of the value. Find these two, label them A, get them done. Leave most of the other eight undone, because the value you will get from them will be significantly less than that of the two highest-value items."[4]

WE INTERRUPT THIS SCHEDULED PROGRAM . . .

Interruptions are probably the greatest bane of carefully planned days, but interruptions will come. Unexpected guests will arrive. Children will get sick. A gabby neighbor will call. We can almost count on at least one change in plans every day.

That's why prayer is so important in Christian planning. It harnesses greater wisdom than our own about what truly matters.

One Sunday afternoon eight years ago, a lanky teenager showed up on my doorstep with a hopeful grin. "I was in the neighborhood," he explained, "and thought I'd come in and wait for services, if that's all right with you." He sniffed. "Do I smell cookies?"

I could have screamed. We worshiped at half-past

four in the afternoon in those days, and my husband had already left to get ready. I was baking cookies (one of my least favorite activities) for a reception after church. In the next hour I had to bake one more batch, wake and change two small boys, and dress myself. "Why now, Lord?" I longed to groan. Instead, with visions of what a hungry teen can do to a dozen cookies, I put on my best preacher's wife smile and said, "Oh sure, come on in."

He started down the hall to the kitchen. "May I help? I just love to make cookies."

In the next hour that young man baked my cookies, woke and dressed the three-year-old, read him a story, and entertained the baby while I dressed. For the first time I knew what Hebrews means when it talks about entertaining angels unaware! Richard came that day as God's interruption, a gift to my life.

Many other interruptions, however, don't feel like gifts. They pump pressure into our lives and sometimes wreck our plans. I can give no pat answer about when they come to provide an opportunity for service and when they come to test our ability to stick to a task without being distracted. I do know from experience that God gives both.

Betty suggested one criterion for making that distinction. She spoke of a time when the busy life of their community caused them to cease daily worship. Since they were founded as a worshiping community, they eventually realized they were out of balance. They discussed the possibility of holding daily worship just before dinner. "We came up with all sorts of objections. What about the children? What about the people fixing dinner? But we knew worship would honor

God, and that was what we were about. Finally we just set our face like flint and decided we would do it, no matter what. God has blessed that. Nowadays it's hard to believe we thought it would be hard."

What most honors God? That question can help us know when we have to decide how to deal with an unexpected interruption to our plans. Sometimes we will make the right choice.

I find that interruptions save me from the myth that I truly control my life. They also make me look forward to an eternal home where nobody interrupts.

EXERCISE

Find more time in your day

1. List everything you do more than four times a week and calculate how many minutes you spend on each per week. Use the chart below to determine how many hours a year you are spending on each task.

Minutes/Day	Minutes/Week	Hours/Year	Eight-Hour Days/Year
5	35	30	3.8
10	70	60	7.6
15	105	90	11.4
30	140	120	15.8
60	280	240	31.6

We see that a daily ten-minute chat consumes the equivalent of seven eight-hour *days* in a year. A five-minute task consumes nearly four eight-hour days!

2. Identify low-value, routine tasks that presently consume what you feel is too much of your

time. What can you do to reduce that time?
(Chapter 11 offers a few tips.) What can you
eliminate? Can you combine some routine tasks
with activities you really want to do instead?
(E.g., pray for missions while waiting in
preschool traffic line; read half an hour daily
while riding an exercise bike; listen to foreign-
language tapes while commuting to work; pay
bills while children do an art project.)

Remember, you are not trying to squeeze minutes,
but to refocus your life to spend more time on what
you most value.

Make a to-do list for the next twenty-four hours

1. Prayerfully consider what you should do this
   day. This first time, include all calendar items
   and routine tasks such as "fix school lunches" or
   "meet with chiefs of staff."
2. What can you drop, delay, or delegate? To
   whom?
3. Determine your *A*, *B*, and *C* priorities.
4. Use the 80/20 rule. Ask, Which items will give
   the most value?
5. Copy final *A* tasks and *B* tasks onto paper or
   Post-it notes.
6. Ask God to take charge of all interruptions in
   your day.

Tips to Make Life Easier

Many simple things can help reduce the stress in our lives. I've included an alphabetical list of some practical tips that have helped me and other women over the years. They may work for you. They may not. I hope that they at least trigger in your own mind some practical steps you can take to reduce stress in your life.

BASKETS

I love baskets! They're inexpensive, pretty, and they organize a multitude of clutter. For instance:

- Have separate laundry baskets for light and dark dirty clothes, to avoid sorting later.
- Place unopened bills in a basket until you are ready to pay them.

- Keep unanswered letters in a basket beside your desk.
- Have a "chore basket" out of which you draw weekly chores.
- Use a basket for coupons in the kitchen or odds and ends on your dresser.
- Use one basket for errand items (see Errands).

BIRTHDAYS

- List birthdays and anniversaries on your calendar on the day you have to mail the card or buy the gift, not the day they happen. One woman makes two notations: one on the actual day and one three to five days earlier indicating "send Ted's birthday card" or "get gift for Sue's birthday."
- "Make a memory" instead of giving a birthday party and gift.[1] Some memories our children have elected were a trip to a museum, dinner at a Japanese steak house, and a day at the county fair.

CLEANING

If it isn't dirty, don't clean it![2] Now that's the most practical tip in the book. Admit it. Sometimes we waste time cleaning things that aren't dirty.

- Two tips from an experienced maid:
    1. If you do floors and beds, the rest looks clean.
    2. You will always clean longest in the room you start in, so start in the room that matters most right now.

- If you do dishes by hand, soak them in hot soapy water while you read a book, take a bike ride, or play a game. They will have almost washed themselves by the time you get back. Remember the 80/20 rule: 80 percent of the dirt is in 20 percent of the house. Clean the 20 percent most often and ignore the rest until it really needs it.
- Separate straightening from cleaning. Put everything away in a room and then clean it. You'll save time.
- Listen to a favorite radio program or tape while you clean.
- Iron in the living room while watching your favorite television show. (My husband irons while he watches sporting events so he will have accomplished something even if his team loses.)

DIRECTORIES

- In a separate phone directory (a small rolodex or notebook), list all doctors' names and phone numbers under D, airlines under A, baby-sitters under B, family members under F, members of a club or group under the name of that group. Then refer to your directory to avoid needing to get out the larger telephone directory when you call frequently used numbers.
- Have one file folder for "Lists and Addresses" into which you put rosters and membership lists for all clubs, schools, church, and co-workers.
- When changing a friend's address or number, note the date of the change. You won't wonder later which is the "new" address.

ENTERTAINING

- Let others bring food to your parties. Then they feel it's their party too. Also, keep it simple. The purpose of a party is for people to have fun, not to show off what you have or can do. (Maxine)
- When asked what you want for a birthday or Christmas, ask for nice candlesticks, tablecloths, or centerpieces. When guests come, you can set a pretty table at a moment's notice.
- Buy candles and pretty napkins whenever you see them on sale.
- Store-bought deli foods with slices of fresh green pepper on top *look* as if you did a lot of work.
- Make-your-own ice cream sundaes are a good, easy party dessert for both adults and children.
- Likewise, ice cream cones are a big hit for school birthday parties if the teacher will let the children eat outdoors. Take your scoop and napkins, pick up ice cream and cones on your way. Easy!

ERRANDS

- Never run one errand when you can run two or three. Never!
- Have an "errand basket" where you deposit *everything* that requires a trip: library books, coupons for the grocery store, letters to mail, shoes to repair. For big items (suits for the cleaner, a car to take to the shop), drop a note into the basket. When you are ready to leave the house, pick up the basket, sort errands by geographical area, and plan your route. (My younger son says, "For dead

items, like a hamster to return to the pet store, ignore this idea.")
• Never make a trip when a phone call will do.

EXERCISES TO REDUCE STRESS

• Set a timer for five minutes, lie perfectly flat on your back with arms beside you. Breathe deeply and—beginning with your toes—relax each muscle in your body. Five minutes of this is roughly equal to a half-hour nap.
• A handout for arthritis patients recommends the following stress-reducing techniques:
  1. For your body: deep breathing, stretching, exercise, a bath, a massage, and proper eating.
  2. For your mind and emotions: talking with a friend, laughing, crying, reading, doing something you love to do.

FLEXIBILITY

• Look for a pleasant use for an unpleasant situation. When the power went out, our older son brought up a candle and a book. "How about ghost stories in the dark?" he suggested. We had a delightful time!
• Consider other options. If you can't do what you planned, what else could you do instead? One night a dinner guest I scarcely knew arrived before Bob got back from the grocery store (and other errands) with the ham I had planned to cook and serve. The guest suggested we just get a bucket of chicken and add it to the salad, veg-

153

etable, and rolls I had already prepared. It was he who first said to me:

A WISE WOMAN KNOWS:
"The problem is usually not the problem itself,
but what you do with the problem."

HOUSEHOLD RECORDS AND OFFICE SUPPLIES

- Set aside a desk or a couple of boxes to hold office supplies and family files. Take inventory to be certain you have all the supplies you need: file folders, pens, paper, tape, scissors, staples, clips. Having to look for items wastes time.
- Income-tax time isn't such a hassle if you keep all receipts, paid bills, canceled checks, and expense accounts in one place all year long. I use an old shortbread tin.
- Use file folders to store insurance records, medical records, product warranties and information manuals, bank-account information, credit-card information, children's records (social security numbers, immunization records, report cards, swimming-lesson certificates).
- If you have more than one bank account, keep a file of "Where the Money Is If We Need It," listing all of the places you have stored money: investment accounts, CD accounts, insurance policies that have cash dividends available, and any other sources of emergency funds. This can save valuable time in case of injury or death.
- Keep all important papers, such as insurance

policies, mortgages, and certificates of deposit in
a bank safety-deposit box to reduce both clutter
and fire risk.

LISTS

- When a big event approaches, make a detailed
  list of everything you have to do and note when it
  must be done. You won't need to worry about the
  event or look at the list until it's time to complete
  the various tasks, but the act of writing it down
  will help you think clearly through all of the steps
  of preparation. (Mary Gene)
- When you have several tasks in one category (fall
  garden chores, house cleaning chores, letters to
  write) list and post them in a prominent place like
  the refrigerator door. As you find spare minutes,
  check the list. Which one item can you accomplish (fertilize the blueberries, write one letter)?
  You may finish the whole list without "making"
  time to do a single task!

MAJOR TASKS

- Try to do unpleasant jobs first, then reward yourself with a more pleasant one. (Bonnie)
- Before a major task, feed the data and problem
  into your mind a few days ahead. Let your sub-
  conscious get to work before you do.
- If small children or a housebound adult are a
  problem, hire a one-time sitter while you work on
  a major task.
- Control interruptions. Arrange with family or co-

workers not to interrupt you and to protect you from phone calls or visitors. Take the phone off the hook if necessary.
- Go where you can't be reached by phone! Empty church classrooms, public libraries, and airport waiting rooms are great study-writing-reading spaces.
- Borrow a friend's house while she or he is at work. My husband has often done that for private retreats.

MAIL

- Don't open junk mail. Almost never!
- Don't even look at mail until you have time to deal with it.

Then process it into five separate categories:

Urgent—Process it at once.
Can wait—Put it into a basket and read it at a designated time.
Bills—Put into the bills-to-be-paid basket until you are ready to pay them.
Read—Place these in the bathroom, bedroom, or wherever you read.
Toss—Discard all junk mail to the recycle or trash pile.

- Set aside one two-hour slot each month to deal with "can wait" items and to answer non-urgent correspondence.
- Whenever possible, answer a letter on the letter itself, copy, and file your copy.

- Pretty postcards can replace short personal letters. Postcards are cheaper to mail, take less time to write, and remove the "guilties" for unanswered correspondence.
- Occasionally evaluate magazines and newspapers. Do you read them? Do they feed your mind or spirit? Cancel subscriptions or have them redirected to someone who will read them.

MEAL PLANNING

- Designate one night a week leftover night.
- The cost of making "impulse" purchases at the grocery store averages one-fourth of most grocery bills. By shopping once a month for primary items, you can save three trips and one week's grocery bill! (The bill seems enormous until you divide it by four.)
- If you have school-aged children, let each child plan one week's menus, or let each child plan a menu for a night he or she will cook. (Commit yourself to eating what is fixed!)
- Start a loose leaf cookbook for each child, giving detailed instructions for making his or her own favorite main dishes, vegetables, and desserts.
- Like ice cream? Save time and calories—make it an entire meal by adding fruit and nut toppings.
- Plan meals that take only a short time to prepare. If something can be eaten in ten minutes, then don't take too much longer than that to cook it. (Gail)
- When having covered-dish or potluck dinners, eliminate dessert. Often people come to the

dessert table groaning, "I really shouldn't eat this." Why waste time preparing foods most people don't think they should eat? (A pastor's wife)

• Clean out recipes you won't ever use and plan to try those you think you want to keep. One new dish a week is fifty-two a year! Alan Lakein warns, "The homemaker who clips another recipe when she has five hundred untried is wasting time."

NOTEBOOKS OR FILES FOR SPECIAL THINGS

• If you like to garden, make a "lawn and garden" notebook, with one page for each month's chores and separate pages for seasonal chores. On facing pages, list supplies (fertilizer, pesticides, seeds) you regularly need that month. Near the beginning of each season and month, check the list and decide when you can do what. Add tips from newspapers and magazines as you read them, so you will know when is the best time to prune azaleas, dig irises, or whatever.

• If you entertain often, keep a file or notebook listing guests, what you fed them, food allergies, and preferences.

• If you enjoy giving gifts, keep a "gift ideas" file. Include in it ideas you pick up from visits or chance remarks such as "I wish I had a . . . ." Also file business cards from craft shows and mail-order catalogues of items you particularly like.

• If you keep a lot of notebooks, consider whether

you are using them to *save* time or fill it. Are there some you really don't need?

PAPERWORK

• Don't deal with a piece of paper twice unless you absolutely must.

SPACES YOU INHABIT

• Think about the items that clutter your living space. Are they items you need? If not, give them away. If you do use them, do they need a space of their own? Do you need to add shelves to closets, hooks to vacant walls, even another closet or storage shed?

• Put items you use most often in the most reachable places, items you seldom use in hard-to-reach places. Anytime you pass or move a seldom-used item to reach an often-used one, you are wasting your time! How far do you reach for a dictionary? Your favorite cookbook? Can you move them closer?

• Designate one drawer the "everything drawer" or "junk drawer."

• Analyze your use of drawers. Are sink utensils nearest the sink, stove utensils nearest the stove? At work, are frequently used office supplies near at hand—or across the room? (No law says you can't have two open boxes of clips in two places.)

• In your closet, put most-worn items in the center, seldom-worn ones on the sides or in back.

- Teach young children to put away their own clothes. For non-readers, tape pictures on the front of drawers to indicate what clothing goes where.
- Eliminate and concentrate. In most of our houses, less is actually more—more space, more air to breathe, more time free from cleaning.[3] Therefore, get rid of *anything* that does not have meaning in your life: clothes you don't wear, books you don't read, records you don't listen to, dishes you don't use, chairs you don't sit on. They are all taking up your space, your air, and your time every time you move them or clean them.

TIME

- Remember: Do what you value! Alan Lakein encourages his readers to ask, What is the most valuable use of my time right now?
- "Shoot while the ducks are flying! Figure out what is most important to do *at that particular time*. Keep asking yourself, What will give me the most satisfaction to do today?" (Martha)
- If it's worrying you, do something about it now, even if it's just to write it on your calendar or to make yourself a note! Worry saps time and energy.
- Reevaluate your television-watching time. Turning off the set may give you lots of time to do other things. (Donna)
- Combine tasks. "I combined my desire to be with my grandson and my desire to help young mothers in our church by beginning a Mothers'

Morning Out each Tuesday. My grandson and I go together to what amounts to a party time for both of us." (Gail)

WAITING TIME

- Waiting time is a gift: you can pray, read, plan.
- Use bits of time to do instant tasks.
- Keep books and magazines in places where you can pick them up when you are waiting: in the car for when you wait for your children to finish sports practice; near the telephone for when you wait "for the next available representative" to take your call; in your purse for when you are on a commuter train, in a doctor's office, in an airport waiting room.
- Waiting time is also a good time to play mini-games with children: "I Spy," "How Many Red Things Do You See?"

WHEN THINGS ARE AWFUL

- Measure this awful time against another you've already endured. I have one hot September night as my standard. We had nine people living in our household—five of them under six years old—and Bob had torn the kitchen down to studs. We were cooking in an upstairs utility room, the refrigerator was still downstairs, and the freezer was in the basement. It was canning season, and the other mother and I stood in that stifling makeshift kitchen all day canning applesauce, tomatoes, blueberries, and kraut. The only time we left was to change diapers, settle quarrels, and put children to bed. Finally, at one o'clock in the morning, we clung to each other and laughed until the tears ran down our cheeks. "It will never get this bad again," we agreed. It never has! And until it does, I refuse to despair.

- Remember: You have to live only this very minute. Do what you have to do in it, then move to the next minute. Don't allow yourself to dwell on "all I have to do," but rather on "what I must do right now."
- Pray. "When I seem to be making bad choices, I remind God that he made me with my gifts and talents. I ask him to help me make good choices." (Shirley)

Tips for dealing with telephones, meetings, procrastination, clutter, and other time wasters that can sabotage our planning efforts appear in the next chapter.

EXERCISE

1. Out of the many ideas discussed in this chapter, list the ones that most appeal to you.
2. Make a list of other stress-reducing ideas you had while you read this chapter.
3. If any of these items need to be entered on a to-do list or calendar, do that now.

CHAPTER TWELVE

Watch Out for Sabotage!

No matter how carefully we plan our days, planning isn't enough. If we truly want to reduce our stress, most of us have to change some habits—especially how we deal with certain saboteurs that waste our time.

TIME WASTERS

Here is one list of Top-Ten Time Wasters:
1. Telephone interruptions
2. Drop-in visitors
3. Meetings
4. Crises
5. Lack of clear objectives, priorities, deadlines
6. Attempting too much in time available
7. Lack of or unclear communication with others
8. Inadequate, inaccurate, or delayed information from others

9. Indecision, procrastination, unfinished tasks
10. Lack of self-discipline.[1]

I definitely would add to the list one more time waster: clutter.

These time wasters eat up minutes and even hours of life unless we take intentional steps to control them. Let's look at a few we haven't mentioned elsewhere.

TELEPHONES

In an earlier chapter we discussed interruptions, which include some phone calls and unexpected visitors. Telephones deserve special mention, however, because they consume such a large proportion of some women's days (including my own).

I love the story of the old Vermonter whose children insisted he put in a telephone. "It's for your convenience," they told him, "so you can call us if you need us."

One day while they were visiting him, the phone began to ring. He didn't move. "Aren't you going to answer it?" his daughter finally asked.

"Nope," he replied. "I got it for my convenience. Now ain't convenient."

Most of us will never get that much control over our telephones, but we can take steps to insure that telephones don't run our lives. If our work includes making or answering calls all day, of course, that's what we will do. When we have calls to make for organizations and clubs, we may use that as time to visit briefly. But, in a day, how many calls that we either make or receive take far longer than they need to? How many calls do we answer or prolong when we need to be doing something else? In the next few days, keep a log of how many minutes you spend on the telephone, then check the chart in chapter 10 for how many hours that is in a year. It may convince you to change your habits!

Telephone Tips

Remember: The telephone is in your house for *your* convenience.

- When you are doing major projects, decide not to answer the phone for a time. Arrange to have calls forwarded to someone else (trade a morning of answering with a friend), use an answering machine, or take the phone off the hook.
- When you are busy and someone asks if you have a minute to talk, answer honestly and gently, "No, I'm afraid I don't right now." Set up a mutually convenient time for a call. When you call other people, make a habit of asking them if this is a convenient time for them to talk.
- Limit your calls. You may want to post a sign near the phone: "Are you talking too long?" (My family suggests posting our last long-distance bill instead.)
- If you must make several calls in a row, list all numbers in one place so that if one phone number is busy or not answering, you can call it later without having to look up the number again.
- Keep a book or handwork near the phone for times when you are placed on "hold."

- You don't have to have a car phone, portable phone, or call waiting just because they're available. Decide for yourself how much of your space and time you want invaded by telephones. Bonnie has a portable phone, which she keeps beside her in the wheelchair. "No more dashing to catch a phone before somebody hangs up!" A great gift for people who are bedridden or in a wheelchair.
- Write elected officials urging a ban on telephone solicitation. Junk mail we can throw away unopened. However, when "junk" phone calls invade our lives, we have to stop whatever we are doing to answer a phone and listen for several seconds to determine that it is a solicitation. (Those who say "You didn't have to answer" obviously don't have relatives who might have an emergency.)

MEETINGS AND OTHER TIME STEALERS

Anybody who has worked with me knows that I loathe meetings—not meetings where something really gets done, but meetings to read minutes, hear financial and committee reports, and deal with issues I have little control over and no interest in. When a meeting drags on, I squirm, chatter about unimportant items, doodle, or even read surreptitiously under the table. So I offer the following.

Tips for More Efficient Meetings

- Define clearly the tasks a meeting is to accomplish. Prioritize the tasks into levels of importance, using the A, B, C method. Handle the A tasks first. Save C items, approval of minutes, and reports until the end if possible.

- Set a time limit for a meeting and stick to it. (Remember: 80 percent of your effectiveness will happen in 20 percent of the meeting anyway!)
- The converse is also true: Honestly budget sufficient time for long agenda items so people know how long the meeting will last.
- If you can put it on paper, do. Allow reading time before or during a meeting. Use agenda time only for questions and approval, not for reading reports and minutes aloud.
- Take time early in the meeting for each person to share briefly about important events or concerns. (Set a time limit for each. Use a timer with a gentle buzzer or beep to let people know their time is up.) This cuts down on extraneous chatter during the meeting itself.
- Never attempt to edit in a committee of the whole. Circulate minutes and documents for individual editing, return to a central person for coordination, and repeat if necessary until you can present to the plenary meeting an almost complete paper for final minor changes.
- Many meetings can be replaced by conference calls, even if the participants live in the same city.

In addition to meetings, other events are notorious time stealers: weddings, funerals, family gatherings, parties, graduation exercises, and volunteer work. All of these can be enjoyable, worthwhile things to do.

They can also waste enormous amounts of time and increase stress if we go out of a sense of duty rather than desire. One rule of thumb: If you feel as bad when you go as when you don't go, don't go!

When holiday traditions overwhelm you, look for time-saving, just-as-pleasant options. One family we know spends each Thanksgiving camping together rather than cooking a huge meal. We serve steak, baked potatoes, and salad for Christmas dinner—the result of one year when we planned to leave for the grandparents' house immediately after dinner and couldn't eat up leftovers. It took so little time to fix that I repeated it the next year, and now it's a firm tradition.

GETTING ADEQUATE INFORMATION

How much life have you wasted because you didn't know exactly when guests were coming, what you were supposed to take to the potluck dinner, or which parts of a job you were supposed to do? Getting the correct information in a timely fashion is critical if we are to use time wisely. It involves:

1. defining precisely what we need to know,
2. determining who has the correct answer, and
3. arranging to get the answer from that person.

That may sound simple, but it can be frustrating. The right person may be out of town or on the telephone all day. That person may have to consult with yet someone else to make a final decision.

Tips for Getting Good Information

• When considering any major undertaking (from

a family Christmas dinner to a corporate
takeover), decide early what you will need to
know from other people and when you can get
the information.

- Put the request in writing well ahead of your
deadline and follow up with a telephone call if
necessary.

- Make it as simple as possible for the other person
to reply: a self-addressed stamped reply card, a
list of options to check, a suggested plan of action
with "Is this okay?"

- If you are uncertain precisely what is required of
you, ask for a written job description for the task.

PROCRASTINATION

A WISE WOMAN KNOWS:
*"Nothing improves procrastination
like the last minute."*

In *You're a Good Man, Charlie Brown*, Charlie lists all
his reasons for putting off writing a book report due
in two days: I'm not really rested, it's not due until
Tuesday, and I work best under pressure anyway.
The charm of his excuses doesn't keep us from identi-
fying with them. Most of us at one time or another
live the adage, "Never do today what you can put off
until tomorrow."

We procrastinate for two primary reasons: the
task looks difficult, or it looks unpleasant. About difficult tasks, Beth said, "One Scripture verse that has
meant a lot to me lately is Isaiah 28:15, 'For we have
made a lie our refuge and falsehood our hiding

place.' I have lived with several wrong beliefs (lies) in my life. One was that anything worth doing had to be done perfectly. I was afraid to fail, so I always put off doing hard things. Writing a letter, for instance, could take me hours, because I wanted it to be exactly right. Jesus is teaching me that I don't have to do everything perfectly. Now I put the dreaded thing first."

Maxine said, "It was my son who taught me, "Mama, what is important is that you *do* it, not that you do it perfectly.'"

Sometimes we procrastinate because we fear we can't do a task at all. We believe we have either too little time or too few skills, and we fear that finally we have bitten off more than we can chew.

Or we may procrastinate because we fear success! A Harvard study of women who showed promise in high school and college but had failed to achieve professional success revealed that women are far more likely than men to avoid success. I don't find that strange. Jesus said if we are faithful in little tasks, we'll be given bigger ones. With all women have to do, who needs bigger tasks?

Unpleasant tasks may be manageable, but we often avoid them because they remind us of former unpleasantness we experienced when we did a similar thing: confronted someone, admitted a mistake, presented a paper nobody praised, cleaned a filthy bathroom, spent hours cooking a meal nobody really appreciated.

Some tasks are both unpleasant and complex. Most of us can put those off until they reach crisis point!

Before discussing some tips about dealing with procrastination, I first want to make a distinction between procrastination and delay. Delay is putting off something until your personal prime time to do it—not filling today with what you don't need to do until tomorrow. For some women, that means delaying a task until several days or weeks ahead of a deadline; for others, it means delaying the task until the day before the deadline. Procrastination means putting off something even past your prime time to do it—looking at that item on your to-do list with fear or loathing and deciding to do something else (several C tasks, for instance) instead.

Tips for Procrastinators

• List reasons you are avoiding a particular job:

— Is it too difficult? Look for one or two easy pieces of it and begin with them.
— Is it unpleasant? What unpleasantness will it entail? How bad will it be? In your mind, walk through the entire unpleasantness. Now ask, How long will the unpleasantness last? Check the clock and start the task, promising yourself, "By such-and-such a time, it will be over!" Or ask yourself, How quickly can I do this if I don't do it perfectly? Set a timer and try to complete it in that length of time.
— Are you afraid you will fail? What is the worst that could happen? Let yourself picture that, then plan what you will do in that case. Once you have made

171

plans to deal with the very worst that could happen, you can get on with the job.
— What is the very best thing that could happen? List positive outcomes and post them where you can see them often as you work.

• Prayerfully consider who else could help you with this. What can you offer in exchange?
• Break large, difficult tasks into big jobs, small jobs, and instant jobs (under ten minutes). Post the list of small and instant tasks where you will see it often, and do one or two as you can.
• Do hard or unpleasant tasks when you are fresh and rested.
• Promise yourself a specific, special reward when you are done. (We will talk more about rewards in chapter 14.)
• Make a deal with yourself: I will work for thirty minutes on this task today, then I may quit if I want to. Set a timer.
• Do unpleasant tasks as if you were a daughter of the King of Kings (and you are!). Langdon Gilkey, in *Shantung Compound*, reports that the only people who would clean filthy prison camp latrines were British aristocrats. Relatives of a king face any task with grace.
• If all else fails, decide to quit. Perhaps this job is not for you after all. Consider all consequences of not doing the task, and if you are willing to face them, turn your back on the task. Do not, however, permit yourself to worry about it afterward.

CLUTTER

Clutter kills! It increases stress, which aggravates heart problems and can lead ultimately to death. Keep that in mind as you read this chapter and look about your home and workplace.

We could pick up each item we own and ask, "Is this worth dying for?" Ruth Volid, a Chicago art dealer, suggested another criterion in an interview with the *Chicago Tribune*: "I keep nothing that has no meaning in my life."

I liked that, especially since we were packing to move at the time. I have found "Does this have meaning in my life?" a marvelous question to ask not only about possessions, but also about groups, relationships, and reading matter. For now, however, let's consider possessions and clutter.

Clutter is too much of anything for the space we have—magazines we don't read, clothes we don't wear, dishes we don't eat on, papers we are done with or will never use, files we don't open, and anything we bought in bulk and don't have room to store.

Clutter wastes life—every time we move it to find something else, every time we have to look for something and can't find it, every time we pack and move it, and every time we clean or dust it.

Clutter is probably the most subtle sabotage in our lives. We know when we procrastinate. But we scarcely notice when we reach past unused glasses to get the ones we want or have to scramble beneath papers on our desk to answer the phone. We get so used to clutter that most of us don't even see it—until we look. One author has written an entire book about clutter.[2]

Tips for Dealing with Clutter

- Straighten the clutter every night, then when you get up, you don't have to face yesterday's clutter. (Shirley)
- Use three headings: "I need," "I want," and "I have." Inventory categories such as shirts, pairs of shoes, televisions, books, records, pots and pans, sets of dishes, whatever. If you have more in any category than you either want or need, give some away. Keep this in mind when making new purchases: Do I need this or even really want it?
- Or inventory one room a month using Volid's question, Does this have meaning in my life? Get rid of anything that no longer has meaning for you. It may be just what somebody else needs.
- Consider creative ways to share the excess. One Christmas my mother gave as gifts things of hers she had heard us admire. Or have a garage sale and give the proceeds to an organization that helps the poor and hungry. Or give the items to a service organization like Goodwill or the Salvation Army, which employs needy people and provides goods at inexpensive prices. Is what you do not need somebody else's necessity?

A WISE PERSON ONCE SAID:
*"The coat hanging unused in your closet
belongs to one who needs it;
the shoes rotting in your closet
belong to the person who has no shoes."*[3]

- If clutter is necessary (as it sometimes is), put it where it won't worry you. Put up a card table for a project, or pile laundry in an unused corner rather than on the sofa or dining table, where you'll have to clear it soon. Then forget about it until you are ready to deal with it.
- Screen off cluttered areas. Maxine kept several large privacy screens when her children were small. If company was coming, she put a screen around various projects. "The size of a party depended on how many screens I had up at the time," she laughs. Her idea could work in some offices too.
- Make a buying rule: for each item you purchase, discard another. Limit how much "stuff" you are willing to live and work with.
- Warning: Make your goals before you clean closets. Otherwise you may throw out just what you're going to need.

TOO-EFFICIENT LIVING

We can live so efficiently that we sabotage our efforts to live effectively. Too much time management can hurt a family, an office, a marriage, or a church. People are important. It's important, therefore, to take time for play as well as work, leisure as well as activity. Sometimes we accomplish the most by doing nothing! Breakfast dates with a spouse or friend, games with children, celebrations with co-workers, parties for a congregation—all of these are life builders, not time wasters. Gloria and her husband take a week each fall at the beach, just to rest, recreate, and refocus their lives and their relationship.

A WISE PERSON ONCE SAID:
"What I look for is not
how to gain a firm hold on myself and on life,
but primarily how to live a life
that would deserve and invoke an eternal Amen." [4]

EXERCISE

1. Out of the many ideas discussed in this chapter, list the ones that most appeal to you.
2. Make a list of other stress-reducing ideas you had while you read this chapter.
3. If any of these items need to be entered on a to-do list or calendar, do that now.

CHAPTER THIRTEEN

A Word About Money

Shirley said, "I want to spend time with my grand-children as they are growing up—take them fishing, buy things for them, travel to see them, bring them to me. That takes money, just as sending four children to college earlier took money. I work in order to earn money. But I always try to remember that it's God's money, just as it's God's time and talents I'm using. They are all given to me to be used in God's way."

Many of our life goals will require money. Travel, education, retirement, even helping others can cost money. Jesus himself needed money to support his ministry (see Luke 8:1—3, noting who paid his bills) and to pay taxes (see Matthew 17).

PUTTING OUR MONEY WHERE OUR GOALS ARE

To be as free from money-related stress as possible, we need to ask, How can the money I spend be directed toward accomplishing my life goals?

Married women will need to decide whether this is a personal or family question. Some families choose to set family goals and direct income toward those. Others may set some family and some personal goals, and provide each person with a monthly allowance to use to meet personal goals.

In the exercise at the end of this chapter, you will be asked to consider which of your goals will require more money than you currently regularly have to spend on them. You could get the money in several ways: steal it, win a lottery, increase income, save in small increments, or redirect spending habits. Since my editors prefer I don't encourage the first two, let's consider the others.

Increasing income means, simply, earning more money. It may involve looking for a higher paying job, changing what you do (which may involve getting more education or training), or, if you aren't earning at all, beginning to earn. A waitress decides to leave a pancake house and seek a job in an elite restaurant because, "If I have to stand eight hours, I might as well earn as much as I can while doing it." A teacher, realizing that her life goal of seeing the world is expensive, decides to leave teaching, return to college, and become a certified public accountant. A mother who wants to send her young children to college decides she must return to work.

Some of those decisions involve a struggle between two goals. If the teacher described above loves teaching, or the mother has a goal of being at home with her children, each must weigh those goals against ones that require more income. Our decisions need not be cut and dried or dreary, but they may still involve some sacrifice. The teacher may look to see where teaching salaries are higher and move, or she may decide to go into administration. The mother may decide to work out of her home or to work only a part-time job.

Sometimes we can pay for a goal in bite-sized pieces. In 1967, I came home from Scotland and got a job where I was earning barely enough to pay bills, but already I yearned to return to Scotland. I asked myself how soon I could go if I saved five dollars a week. The answer, in those days, was two years. Each week I took out my tithe money and my Scotland money first, then lived on the rest. It became such a habit that I have seldom been without a "Scotland fund" since. When I meet people who say wistfully, "I wish I could afford to do such and such," I say, "You can—it just may take you a while."

Saving may involve redirecting what we spend for. One woman looked for a way to save and saw how much she habitually spent at fast-food restaurants, so she decided to keep frozen pizzas, pounds of hamburger patties, and other instant dinners at home. Another woman looked at insurance premiums and decided she could save money by taking a higher annual deductible. A third woman's family moved into a smaller house to buy a boat.

Libraries and bookstores have financial-planning

books that can help you take a realistic look at your finances and decide how you can begin to save toward desired goals.[1]

THE HIGH COST OF MONEY

Sometimes we may want to re-evaluate our entire lifestyle. Every time I see a bumper sticker proclaiming that shopping is a feminine sport, I want to get on a soapbox and shout, "Don't you know that's an advertiser's lie?"

Until World War II, women were co-producers with men. At home, women spent long hours providing food and clothing for households. On farms and in factories, women worked as hard as men, although sometimes at different tasks. During the war many of them took over traditionally male jobs while men went to the battlefields.

When the war ended, men again replaced women in the work force. At the same time, new labor-saving devices made "women's work" easier. No longer co-producers and largely excluded from the work force, what should women be? Madison Avenue had an idea: Let women be consumers! Men will produce goods, women will buy them. Men will earn money, women will spend it. Separate but equally important roles—for the economy, anyway.

If you don't believe me, read old magazines. Until about 1947, ads aimed at women were for clothing patterns and household items, and recipes were for nourishing meals. After the war, ads switched to glamor items. Women were urged to buy manufactured clothes and make themselves party wraps, to buy prepackaged foods and try recipes for gourmet dishes. Later ads returned to "necessities," but sold them as glamor products to help us become "perfect" housekeepers. Current ads for clothes, cosmetics, and even detergents offer to make us look like, or free us to become, rising executives—whether or not we want to!

Don't get me wrong. I don't want to sweat over a wood stove or wring out laundry any more than you do. Low-maintenance houses and more income can free women to do what we feel God wants us to do. The trick is making certain we actually get to do what God wants us to do rather than getting trapped into working long hours to buy what *producers* want us to buy.

"I work because I have to!" you may protest indignantly. It is certainly true that many women get up and go to work every morning simply to put groceries on the table. Our nation is increasingly split between growing sectors of "the very rich and the rest of us."[2]

On the other hand, one reason it often takes two incomes to support a family these days is that "support" includes buying so much. If we were content with 1967 standards for homes and cars, they would cost less in real dollars today than they did then! It is power seats, power windows, cruise control, tilt steering wheels, digital clocks, air conditioners, garbage disposals, wall-to-wall carpet, and two-and-a-half baths that we are exchanging our labor—and our lives—for.[3]

The morning I was preparing to mail this manuscript, our local paper carried the story of a banker who was recently laid off. Her salary was $56,200, ". . . 60 percent of our household income. This was not for luxuries and ballet classes," she lamented, "it was for mortgage payments, car payments, and the necessities of life. Unfortunately we were terrible savers, so we have no cushion."[4] Is it really possible to spend $100,000 a year purely on "necessities"?

Yes, if luxury is a necessity. It is not coincidence that as women have returned to the workplace, yesterday's upper-class lifestyle has become the middle-class norm. Manufacturers introduce new cosmetics, personal care products, designer clothes, and "toys" for men, women, and children at a dizzying rate. In 1980, how many of us wanted—much less needed—a microwave oven, personal computer, VCR, video camera, Jacuzzi, hot tub, cellular phone, answering machine, portable phone, Walkman radio, jogging suit, digital watch, membership in a health club, designer clothes, or Nintendo? By 1990, a scant ten years later, how many of them did we have? Dividing the price of each item by the hourly income earned in our family, how many hours of life did each cost? (On how many of them did we pay credit-card interest rates?)

I have a theory about one part of our high consumption—the amount we spend on children. In 1959, a new "necessity" was created for little girls: Barbie dolls. When Barbie was introduced, psychologists worried that little girls were being encouraged to identify with a teenager. But little girls don't identify with dolls, they mother them. Is it any wonder that little girls who mothered the world's most consumptive teen grew up to be real life mothers willing to buy designer baby clothes and send children to college with microwaves and refrigerators?

To me, one of the saddest sights in contemporary America is a community of enormous houses standing empty five days a week while everybody goes to work in order to pay for the houses. On Saturdays the families clean and do yard work, and on Sunday they crash. No wonder! When an expensive, gorgeous house is the god, staying home on Sunday is an appropriate form of worship. But when do families really enjoy those homes? Are the houses worth the lifetimes that go to pay for them?

People who don't know me well may think I'm urging women to stay home while men go out to work. Not at all! I know women who stay home and run up enormous bills that their husbands are literally killing themselves to pay.

In a perfect world, we would use our income to enhance our lives and reduce our stress. In this world, money-related stress is consuming whole families. Therefore, I urge women to look at both their personal and their family goals and revise their spending habits to support, not sabotage, those goals.

NEW WAYS TO SPEND

Several years ago a friend told me about prayerful shopping: praying as you browse, "God, give me wisdom to spend your money wisely." I tried it, and I've discovered that it works. I now buy far less and more wisely. I find myself less impressed by brand names than by quality goods, less impressed by new products than by secondhand ones with a lot of life still left in them, less prone to buy something just because everybody else has one.

Other questions that make us wiser shoppers are:

1. How many working hours does this cost my household? Is it worth that many hours of life to me?

2. What is its cost per use? Sometimes buying a more expensive item that lasts longer is cheaper if you plan to use or wear it for a while.

3. Am I buying this item because I truly want or need it—or because I'm bored or depressed and have a charge card in my pocket? If the latter is true, what is a wiser or cheaper alternative?

Bonnie prays as she writes monthly checks, thanking God for whatever she is paying for and praying for those who receive each check. "An attitude of gratitude lets me enjoy some purchases twice and notice blessings that aren't so visible."

"Tithing is a discipline that seems to order the rest of our lives," Gail said. Several women related tithing to an ordered life. Our own children resisted tithing their incomes at first, but we keep telling them that if they get used to giving God ten percent of ten dollars, it won't hurt as much later to give God ten percent of ten million!

THE HOLE OF DEBT

Debt is a big, deep hole that consumes energy, wealth, health, sanity, and the future. We get into debt because what we want right now, or think we deserve, is more than we can afford except by mortgaging our future. My observation is that men go into debt for big items—leasing a car, buying a time-share unit at the beach—while women go into debt for designer jeans, shoes on sale, and fast-food evenings when we don't want to cook. When I look at my credit-card bills some months, I want to gasp, "Those little purchases couldn't have totaled this much!"

A WISE WOMAN KNOWS:
*"It's less painful to be swallowed by an alligator
than to be nibbled to death by ducks."*

Taking control of our lives means taking responsibility for our debts. No matter how well we state goals and plan our days, if our debt service (what it costs each month to pay credit cards, mortgage, and other loans) eats up most of our income, we're going to live under stress.

One of our first A-priority goals, therefore, needs to be either to pay our debts or to unload any items we are buying on time and get no satisfaction from owning. We have little chance of channeling money toward other goals until we achieve that one.

There are several ways to accomplish this. One woman said, "I bit the bullet, cut up my charge cards, and set aside money to pay my debts out of each pay check right after I took out my tithe. Tithing and paying my debts were my A-number-one priorities that year." Another woman calculated how long it would take her to pay off her credit cards and automobile loan if she worked two jobs, taking a second job only for that duration. Another family discovered that refinancing their home was a good way to consolidate all their debts: the new mortgage interest rate was far less than interest rates on their credit cards and automobile loans, and they could use the money from the mortgage to pay off the higher interest loans immediately.

For many people, however, getting out of debt is a problem for experts. Financial-planning workshops and personal-investment counselors can help calculate how soon we can pay debts and begin to move toward other goals.

EXERCISE

1. Determine which of your goals will require money. How much money will they require?
2. How will you get the money? When will you get it?
3. Revise your annual and monthly goals to include making or saving money toward your goals.
4. If debt or poor planning are part of your situation, what steps will you take to get out of debt? When will you take them?

CHAPTER FOURTEEN

Coping in a Less-Than-Perfect World

I once knew a young mother with a knack for wise sayings. When she arrived late with preschool children, she said, "If you only knew how early I started to get here this late." Another saying was, "The world stops for dirty diapers."

Some authors of "how to manage your time" books write as if we could, by our own efforts, create a perfect world. "Handle each sheet of paper only once," they advise. "Make all your calls in the first half hour of the day." Those writers correctly assume that many stresses come from a lack of organizational skills. But what about the rest of the stress?

For most of us, our world has to stop every day for dirty diapers or some equivalent. People we call aren't home and have to be called again. Letters we want to write require further research and have to be laid aside. Unexpected deadlines overlap with deadlines we were already struggling to meet. Friends have a personal crisis. Bikes get stolen. Fillings fall out. Loved ones drastically disappoint us—even die. Accidents happen.

In addition to organizational skills, therefore, women must also develop a repertoire of techniques that can help us cope with the stress of living in an imperfect world.

GIVE YOURSELF PERMISSION TO . . .

Gloria, a Christian marriage and family therapist, peppered our interview with the term "give myself permission." I asked what she meant.

"We are often bound by words like *should* and *should not*," she replied. "Women are not given permission by society to think, to be powerful or strong, to take charge of our lives, so we don't. We are given some permission to cry, but often we feel guilty about our tears and try to choke them back. Also, because they reveal many different emotions—fear, guilt, sadness, anxiety, anger, PMS, or even joy and tenderness—our tears confuse the males in our lives. It helps if we can clarify to them verbally what our tears mean. I manage to do this about three quarters of the time now, and my husband has learned he does not have to 'fix' my tears, because he is usually not responsible for them. I have also given myself permission to be angry with God at times. I have discovered God can deal with that."

Nancy also spoke of how it relieved her tension to know God could deal with her anger toward a God who could permit her husband to die. Bonnie spoke of the freedom that comes when we give ourselves permission to cry.

Gloria concludes, "I try to help women give themselves permission to become and do what they want to become and do."

As we seek prayerfully to limit what we do, and thereby reduce stress in our lives, we need to give ourselves permission to ask what we do not need to do, and what is causing the most stress. We need to give ourselves permission to feel angry, scared, and powerful. We even need to give ourselves permission to grow!

A WISE WOMAN KNOWS:
"Nature does not demand perfection; It only requires that we grow."[1]

TAKE TIME TO BE HOLY

When C. S. Lewis was an atheist, he was surprised that many of his favorite authors were Christians. At first he considered each a great writer "in spite of that," but gradually he had to admit that it was their faith that gave them depth and appeal.[2]

Similarly, I discovered that women who cope well with stress seem to have one major thing in common: all rely heavily on prayer, most have daily Bible study as well. That is certainly not true for all Christians. A study of how faith begins and grows found that few religious professionals or laypeople can articulate what prayer actually does to their faith; even fewer regularly open the Bible for personal study.[3]

Why are regular times of prayer and Bible reading

so hard for most of us? Is it because we are used to thinking of prayer and Scripture study as something we "must" do—a boring duty or discipline? Is it because we think it could be wonderful but seems self-indulgent in the middle of everything else we simply must get done? Or is it because we simply don't know how to spend half an hour in Scripture reading and prayer, so have found our few attempts arid and not very relevant to the rest of life?

The women I spoke with said (and my own experience is) that we begin to pray and study daily when it becomes not a chore or a luxury but the most important part of the day—a re-fueling, an oasis, a time of joy and self-discovery. Betty, speaking of her personal devotions and two daily community worship times, says, "They frame my life and give structure to it."

One attitude change that helped me develop a more regular habit of prayer was when I began to consider regular prayer and Scripture study as a goal, not a commitment. Putting "pray and study four times a week" on my goals list lets me measure how well I have done and strive to do even better, whereas making a commitment and failing to meet it used to make me feel guilty.

We must, of course, give ourselves permission to "deserve" half an hour or more a day to build our spirits without also feeling guilty about shutting out family, co-workers, and telephones. When we do, however, families and offices do not fall apart—quite the reverse. Beth spoke of taking a "prayer break" each afternoon just before her four children come home from school. "Sometimes when I get frazzled, the children beg, 'Mama, take another prayer break!'"

Ann writes, "If I begin my day with half an hour or more of Bible study, prayer, and reading someone like Oswald Chambers, Henri Nouwen, C. S. Lewis, or any number of others, then I don't go into my day feeling as if the gun to start the race has sounded and I had better run for all I'm worth. If I don't start out with a clear focus and communication with the Lord, then I'm very likely to allow the stress that is certainly there to become overwhelming. Those parts of a Christian's life are so basic, so obvious, so essential. How can a Christian who has known the joy of them ever get lax? I don't know how—but I know it's easy and I also know it's deadly."

Sometimes we may have to settle for less-than-best during different seasons of life. One mother of three children under age six reads her children a Bible story daily and prays with them, and counts it her own prayer time, too. "In a few years I'll get back to my own time, but this is the best I seem to be able to do just now," she says. Donna, an early riser, always had her time of prayer and study in the early morning before making hospital rounds. Now, however, her preschool son likes to rise as soon as she does. "No matter how quiet I am, he hears me and comes padding in. I used to get up at half-past five, then five o'clock. When we were both getting up at half-past four, I realized this just wasn't going to work. Now I play with him in the mornings and have my prayer time in the evenings. It's not as good because I'm worn out, but I keep reminding myself that this is temporary. One day he'll sleep later, and I'll get mornings back."

Donna also speaks to women who don't know

where to begin Scripture study. "I'm currently working on a program to read the Bible in a year. It calls for me to read three chapters of Old Testament and one of New Testament each day, with a psalm and a chapter of Proverbs every third day. Seeing how slowly I'm progressing, it'll probably take me three years, not one, but I refuse to let myself get stopped by that. I don't feel guilty that I don't get as much read as the program suggests. Instead, I enjoy what I read and know that at the end of a week I've read a lot more than I would have otherwise."

I personally have a different system. Persuaded that our Lord is a great teacher who knows me better than I know myself, years ago I began asking him to direct my Scripture reading. Each time I complete one book of Scripture, I run my eyes down the Bible's table of contents and pray, "What now?" When my eye stops at one particular book, that's what I read.

As I begin to read, I ask, "What would you have me see?" Then I read slowly, like savoring a favorite food. If something catches my eye, I pay even more careful attention to it. Sometimes I read a book that I know little about (Haggai, for instance) and discover a new truth (in that case, a person—the great layman Zerubbabel). Sometimes I find answers to precisely the questions I have been asking. And sometimes I find so little there that I have to go back and ask, "What did you want me to see here, Lord?" Then a verse, concept, or repeated word rises from the page to teach me a truth I didn't realize I needed to know.

One thing that makes a prayer habit easier is having a special chair where you regularly go to pray, a place where your Bible, prayer concerns notebook, and perhaps a devotional book are in easy reach. When we have to look for our Bible and decide where and when to sit each day, the habit is harder to develop.

For those who have not yet developed a prayer habit and feel guilty about starting only when life is unmanageable, Oswald Chambers says (translated for women), "When a woman is at her wits' end, it is not a cowardly thing to pray. It is the only way she can get into touch with Reality. Be yourself before God and present your problems, the things you know you have come to your wits' end over."[4]

In chapter 6 we looked at the purpose for each of our lives. "Continually restate to yourself what the purpose of your life is. The destined end of women is not happiness, nor health, but holiness."[5] Daily seeking that holiness is one major step toward coping with the stress of an imperfect world.

REST WHEN YOU'RE WEARY

A surprising number of women I interviewed declared that getting enough sleep is essential for them to maintain low-stress lives.

"Sometimes I nap," Gail admitted. "On occasion, I just quit!"

"Balancing rest, private space and time, and spiritual feeding with whatever else I'm doing is crucial," said Martha.

Maxine refuses stimulants like the caffeine in coffee, tea, and chocolate after three o'clock in the afternoon, because she needs to get to bed by half-past nine in order to rise at three o'clock in the morning. Then she naps when she gets home from work before setting out on her other commitments.

"Getting enough sleep is essential for me," declared Helen. "I need seven hours of sleep a night, at least, and sleeping enough is a real matter of spiritual discipline for me. I tend to try to do more and more before I go to bed. But when I do that consistently and don't get the rest I need, a shade of separation comes down. I shift into overdrive, concentrate on getting tasks done, and ignore people around me. My husband says I lose all my softness around the edges."

While half the world gears its schedule to a daily siesta, we live in a society where mothers even boast, "My child never naps." My response (usually silent) is, "Poor child!" Most children will nap if their mother reads them a story, rocks them, puts them down at the same time every afternoon for several days, and leaves them in quiet for a couple of hours. My own two children napped for one simple reason: their mother needed a nap! I used to feel guilty about my nap habit—especially after the children entered school. But I know it's one thing that helps keep me sane. I was considerably relieved to hear other women say they nap too, and I always rejoice when a new study indicates that naps can significantly lower stress levels and should be part of our lifestyle. Let's give ourselves permission to get enough rest!

Another way to rest is to observe the weekly sabbath. God doesn't *suggest* we take one day apart for rest and holiness; he *commands* it. After my husband researched and delivered a sermon about observing

the sabbath, we began to set aside Sunday afternoons for rest, recreation, and re-creation of our spirits. We give ourselves permission to nap, laze
around, or go to the beach; we do no chores, usually
eat out after church, and even though both of us
have offices at home, we do not go to our desks. The
discipline of that means we have to work harder
other days of the week. (I rose this morning at 6:45
on a *Saturday*, for instance, to complete the final
draft of this book, for it must be mailed Monday,
and I will not work on it tomorrow.) We find that
knowing we will rest one day a week orders the rest
of our schedule.

Gordon MacDonald in *Ordering Your Private World*
says that since he preaches Sunday mornings, he and
his wife observe a Tuesday sabbath instead. If you
must must work on Sunday, what other day of the
week can you substitute as your God-given day of
rest?

NOW GET OUT THERE AND RUN!

Most women I interviewed have some form of exercise each week—putter in the yard, play tennis, walk,
run. Whatever they do, they spoke of the importance
of exercise in reducing stress.

"I have to keep a balance in my life," says Donna.
"The hard necessity for me is to take care of my physical person. I don't really enjoy exercise [You could
have fooled me—she's one of the most consistent jog-
gers and swimmers I know] but if I don't do it, I get
out of whack mentally and spiritually. My work suffers too. I've joined a fitness center and swim three or

four times a week. I also have a tendency toward weight problems, so I watch what I eat."

"I do regular exercises," says Gloria, "and I walk almost every morning. As I walk, I pray over my day—for the people I plan to see and how God is leading me to relate to them. At night I swim for half an hour and hand it all over to God until the next day."

I personally have never been fond of exercise. To and from the refrigerator for another glass of tea is my preferred daily quota. I even teased my mother-in-law about her three-times-a-week aerobics class. But when she had a serious automobile accident, she made a rapid, amazing recovery. Doctors said again and again, "It's because she was in such good shape."

When my husband moved to Florida a couple of months before the rest of the family, he began to take daily long bike rides. When we got to Florida, we found him so slim and fit that he inspired the rest of us! We got our bikes in shape the week we arrived, and all summer as I wrote this book, we also took at least one long bike ride and one evening at the beach each week. Other nights we strolled around the neighborhood or went to a pool for laps. I hate to admit it, but I was able to think more clearly, sleep more soundly, and work at least as many hours as before. Can my days as a desk potato be over?

USE GOD'S CHILD-REARING MODEL

Gail admitted that one stress for her was worry that her four children would misbehave. "If they did, I felt so guilty. I worried that maybe I had been away too often, that if I'd been there more they would have learned better behavior." Since I've had those worries (and suspect some of you have, too), I asked what she did about that.

"A variety of things. Sometimes I pulled back and spent more time with them. Sometimes I admitted that misbehaving is normal. Once our family went to a healing service at an Episcopal church when we felt our teenagers were too hard to manage. I also felt it was very important to help them find good things to do, to keep them so busy with good things they didn't need to look for other things. The church and extra-curricular activities at school took much of the family's time, but we didn't mind." Apparently not—she and her husband were once co-president of the high school PTA and served as counselors of their church youth group for twenty years!

That reminds me of a sermon I once heard. Apparently God never told Israel what *not* to do without telling them what they *could* do instead. A good way to raise our own children too!

ACCEPT YOUR LIMITATIONS

To hear women talk, you would think that most of our stress comes from the demands of other people. When women get honest, however, we admit that much of our stress comes from within, from our unrealistic expectations of ourselves. Therefore, we can eliminate a good bit of stress by accepting who we are and what we can realistically do.

Donna said, "I have high aspirations and goals I have bought into. But sometimes I have to tell myself,

'That will have to wait. I have a whole lifetime. I don't have to do everything at once.' I have gotten into the habit of asking, What am I called to do today? I ask it once emphasizing 'today,' then I have to ask it emphasizing 'I'—so I don't get stressed out trying to make my husband, son, or co-workers do what I think they should be doing! I have to let go of what is not mine to do."

Maxine said, "I have to avoid spreading myself too thin. I don't accept jobs that I can't do well. Avoiding leadership avoids stress for me, so I don't chair too many committees at once. And I don't resent what I have to do. If I have agreed to do it, I find ways to do it. I find that being positive and having a sense of humor helps a lot." (Wide smile.)

Betty said, "I've had to learn to be content without having my finger in every pie, to live without desiring to control my husband and my children. De-stressing my life has involved entrusting to other brothers and sisters things that really matter to me and that affect my life."

Shirley said, "Over the years I've learned to leave things I can't deal with to God. If I can't do anything about something, I refuse to spend time worrying about it."

Helen said, "My greatest stress comes when I underestimate my own physical abilities and limits on my time—sign on for more than can physically be done in the time I have to do it. Being newly married, I find, requires time and emotional energy. Relationships that are what we want them to be take a lot of time."

Bonnie said, "When I hear myself telling myself

'I should have . . . ,' I stop and remind myself that I've been doing the best I could. If I took time out to read or watch television, I needed to do that. If I've really wasted time, I forgive myself and move on. I also remember that what is, is. I once heard someone say that when we resist what is, we are living in hell. Some things in life are given. For me: this wheelchair, singleness, too much to do. If I resist those things, life becomes far more stressful than if I accept them and get on with what I am able to do."

REWARD YOURSELF

Donna first suggested this concept to me. "Some disciplines—exercising, eating right—give me a sense of well-being that is its own reward. But I struggle with procrastination. For big jobs that I keep putting off and maybe didn't really want to do anyway, doing a good job is not enough. Then I give myself specific rewards. *Big* rewards, not little ones like food, that soon disappears and contributes to another problem.

"One day I sat down and listed some of the unmet needs in my life. Two are a need to build up my self-esteem and a need to be really heard and loved. When I was growing up, I often wore hand-me-down clothes, so one thing that builds up my esteem is really looking good.

"When I do a big job—writing a paper to present at a midwives' conference, for instance—I reward myself for the hard work by buying myself a really nice outfit to present it in. Or if I make it through a period with lots of babies to deliver, I reward myself with a visit to my therapist for one hour of unconditional caring and listening.

"Women spend a lot of time nurturing and caring for others. I think it's important for us to nurture and care for ourselves too."

Elise echoed this theme. "I give myself three rewards for accomplishing all I do every day. First, I get my nails sculptured every three weeks. That seems silly to some people, but I have always bitten my nails. As a lawyer, my hands are in public view all day long, and my nails were a source of constant embarrassment. Now it's such a treat to have pretty nails. That both rewards me and removes one cause of stress. I also play tennis each week, twice sometimes—three times is heaven! And since I spend so much time in my car, I bought myself a gorgeous and very comfortable one. It feels like a cocoon to me at times."

Both these women are executives with high-pressured jobs and good salaries. Obviously the rewards they give themselves differ from what others would or could choose. But several women named ways they reward themselves for hard work. Shirley goes fishing. Maxine goes shopping—driving twenty miles to another town so she doesn't run into anybody who wants to talk. "I don't necessarily buy anything on those days. I just wander around." Travel is another reward for her—and a great incentive to get work done. "I tell myself, 'I want to get this much done before we go.'"

I found the whole idea of deliberately rewarding oneself intriguing. Since most of what I do is what I enjoy doing, I presumed that for myself, doing a task is reward enough. Or is it?

No. I realized there are some Saturdays after a rough week when I announce, "I'm spending the morning in bed with a book," mornings when I finish a chapter and join Bob for a cup of tea, lunchtimes when I meet somebody for an hour in the middle of a deadline, and many evenings when I decide, "I've worked too hard today to have to cook." And because somebody else may tell you if I don't, I was well known in one office for my three o'clock Snickers break! Perhaps some of us reward ourselves unconsciously!

Call it reward or celebration, one sure way to reduce stress in our lives is to balance hard work with rewards, things we must do with things we truly want and enjoy.

IN ALL THINGS GIVE THANKS

I was at first surprised and then amazed at how often the word "grateful" flowed from the lips of women I interviewed. Gail mentioned being thankful for a house that is easy to clean, a husband who supports her many volunteer activities, his job that frees him every evening, God's presence with her during the illness and death of her younger son, her church with all its possibilities for ministry, people who have picked up projects she started and have helped them grow, positions she has been "privileged" to have in various community organizations, and her congregation. She even said at one point, "I'm so grateful that we were permitted to work with the young people in our church for many years. We learned so much."

Bonnie echoed the same theme: "When I begin to feel stress, I work on developing and nurturing an attitude of gratitude. I find myself thanking God for little things I usually take for granted: flush toilets, running water, air conditioning and heat, carpets on my floor, a pillow beneath my head. As I thank God for these blessings, others come to mind. I spent last week praising God for my ancestors. I find that when I make a deliberate decision to be grateful rather than to complain, stress begins to unravel. If we dwell on problems, we become people with problems—maybe even become problems ourselves! I would rather become a thanksgiving."

Betty's mother, another Betty known as Bey, is past ninety and is one of my dearest friends. She bubbles with gratitude and praise. To be in her presence is to feel you have blessed her just by your existence, and to hear her constant gratitude is to be reminded of blessings you had forgotten you had.

Betty said, "Mother is a living example that order springs out of a life of giving thanks to God. Thanksgiving transforms daily chores and menial tasks that can otherwise be so drab and boring. Truly if there is one thing Bey Carr has given the world, it is an example of a thankful heart."

EXERCISE

1. Are there areas in your life where you need to give yourself permission to:
   grow?
   be weak? (cry about a situation or event?)
   be strong? (take charge of some part of your life?)

give up doing something?
begin to do something you have never done
before?

Choose one area and decide on one thing you will
do today to demonstrate that you have given yourself
permission in that area.

2. Accomplishing a goal of spending regular time
with God requires planning. Do you need to set
up a prayer place? Buy a Bible translation you
enjoy reading? Find a prayer notebook and pen?
Select one or two books for devotional reading?
What can you do today to begin to meet your
own goals in this area?

3. Look at your upcoming day and week. Have
you provided time for rest—a nap, half an hour
with a good book, a few minutes of quiet? Do
you want to exercise? When and how will you
do that?

4. If clamoring children create stress for you, do
they need help in knowing what to do? Would a
little time now devoted to their schedule and
equipment reduce both your stress and theirs?

5. Go back to the exercises in chapter 1 and make a
new stress list. Hopefully many of your former
stresses have been reduced or eliminated. Do
you have some stress now because you have not
accepted your own limitations? Consider your
new stress list and prayerfully let go of: trying
to control other people; things you don't do
well; worry about things you cannot do anything about; anger at yourself for past failures.

One woman suggests this prayer: "Lord, I admit
that I know I am not superwoman. Forgive me for act-

ing like I am. Show me what you want me to do, and what you want me to lay aside. Thank you for accepting me just as I am. Amen."

6. What really rewards you for work well done? What will you do this week to reward yourself for meeting your goals?

7. Consider starting today to practice an "attitude of gratitude." Can you list ten things for which you are grateful? Twenty? Fifty? Can you share that gratitude with others in each conversation you have today? Can you share it with God?

In Summary

Many women do too much—because it makes us feel important or needed or because we believe we must. We have come to believe that if we do not do everything, some pieces of our world will fall apart. That, however, is a myth. God did not create us to do "too much," and prayerful assessment and planning can reduce what we do to a manageable, even enjoyable load.

Our lives, however, will never be free from worry, tension, or stress. Our task as daughters of a loving God is to seek God's best purpose for our lives and steer ourselves in that direction. When we encounter stress, then, we can see it as
- a test God has put in our path,
- an interruption we are supposed to stop and deal with, or
- a sign that we are off course and need to reconsider our direction.

We order our lives and reduce stress by dismantling the barriers to order; by prayerfully setting life goals; by directing our time and our finances toward meeting our goals; and by regularly taking time to rest and refresh our bodies and spirits.

Ultimately, we order our lives and manage stress by turning to the One who made us. On my computer monitor I keep a prayer that Eleanor Roosevelt is reported to have carried in her purse: "Our Father, who has set a restlessness in our hearts and made us all seekers after that which we can never fully find, keep us at tasks too hard for us, that we may be driven to Thee for strength."

As my son Barnabas reminds us, "God says, 'You think you got stress? I order the universe!'"

Surely we can trust One with that much experience to order our lives too.

APPENDIX A

Sample Goals

I've listed here two examples that show how life goals break down into long-term, short-term, annual, monthly, and weekly tasks. Each example also includes what might appear on a daily to-do list. These are only examples, not suggestions for your own life goals!

Life Goal I:
To learn to know, love, and trust God.

This Season's Goal:
    To develop a regular habit of Bible study and
        prayer.

One-Year Goal:
    To pray and study my Bible four times a
        week; to read four books to help with
        spiritual growth in this year.

Annual Plans:
> To set up a place and time for regular prayer
> and study. To choose books to study.

Monthly Tasks In Sequence:
> Check calendar to select best time (Jan.)
> Look at house to select best place (Jan.)
> Choose a Bible translation I like (Jan.)
> Buy prayer notebook (Jan.)
> Select one scripture book to study (Jan.)
> Choose book for growth (February, May,
> August, November)
> Gradually build up to desired frequency of
> prayer/study.
> Evaluate monthly to see how well I have met
> the goal.

One Week's Tasks:
> Set aside four times this week for
> prayer/study.
> Prayerfully choose a translation and one book
> of Scripture to study; begin.

To-Do List for One Day:
> Buy a Bible and a prayer notebook.
> Spend thirty minutes in prayer and study.

Life Goal II:
To make and cherish lasting friends.

This Season's Goal:
> To rekindle old friendships.

One-Year Goal:
> To reestablish contact with college friends I
> haven't seen in years.

Annual Plans:
> To contact three former roommates and
> suggest a small autumn reunion
> on campus.

Monthly Tasks in Sequence:
> Call each to ascertain interest (March).
> If interested, determine a place and time
> (March).
> Plan details: food, travel, fun (summer).
> Attend reunion (autumn).
> Evaluate, consider value of annual time
> together (December).

One Week's Tasks
> Make calls (set aside one or two evenings).
> If they are interested, reserve location.
> Send written confirmation to everyone.

One Day's To-Do Entries:
> Locate phone numbers for each.
> Call Heidi and Masako.
> Buy stationery.
> Buy stamps.

APPENDIX B

Women Who Shared

Ann is a college professor of English, a wife, and the mother of two grown daughters. She is very active in her local church and in the Cursillo movement. Ann also takes other people's small children home with her to give the children a treat and the parents a break. Both her own daughters developed juvenile diabetes when they were young, so their lives have included "shots, food restrictions, blood and urine tests, and emergency rooms." Ann and I have been close friends and prayer partners since high school, and I've watched her balance incredible schedules with humor and common sense.

Beth is a full-time wife and mother of four, ages eight to eighteen. She chooses to invest herself in her marriage, her children, and—as the wife of a seminary professor—seminary wives. At a conference recently, we spoke between interruptions by her children and their friends. Beth gave each child a hug or a word of special encouragement: "I haven't seen that blouse before." "I like the way you're doing your hair." It was obvious that all the children, not just her own, flock to Beth for love and a touch. Her stress—and grief—have been increased recently as two sisters have become chronically and critically ill. Beth has spent much of her time helping to care for them and their seven small children, as well as her own.

Betty, an accomplished musician and composer, is part of a worship team that conducts renewal workshops for local churches in this country and abroad. She also served on the Episcopal church's Standing Committee on Church Music. She and her late husband, the Reverend Graham Pulkingham, were founding members of the Community of Celebration, a religious order located in the Episcopal diocese of Pittsburgh. The community includes twenty-four persons, married and celibate, who for nearly twenty-five years have shared their lives and income and served God in Texas, Colorado, England, Scotland, and now in Pennsylvania. She and Graham raised six children, three of whom are now married. She graciously gave me one morning of her vacation for this interview, then fed me lunch!

Bonnie is part of a three-person community devoted to Christian-education ministry. She uses her master's degree in education to help develop church-school curricula. She also manages the office and carries full responsibility for planning and leading Sunday-morning activities while the rest of the team travels to workshops. Bonnie had polio when she was seven and lives in a wheelchair, so she works and lives alone in a house carefully planned and renovated to accommodate her lifestyle and to minimize stress.

Donna is a Ph.D. nurse-midwife in private group practice. She and her husband, also a nurse, have a four-year-old son. In addition to nursing, Donna loves music; for years she directed the music ministry of her local congregation. When her son was two, Donna's husband had surgery for a malignant brain tumor and had to give up—temporarily, at least— dreams of going into business for himself as a maker of fine handcrafted furniture. This decision plus a staff shortage at work delayed their having another child—adding yet one more stress.

Elise is a lawyer, the wife of a college president, and the mother of three children. Her youngest had just left for college when we spoke; her oldest is currently in law school, about to follow her mother's profession. Elise sits on the board of a seminary and two national Christian ministries. As a break from her exhausting schedule, Elise cherishes a group of five women who meet bimonthly to share, pray, and feed each other gourmet lunches served in style.

Gail met me for lunch less than two weeks before her daughter's wedding and the week after the birth of her third grandchild, yet she seemed her usual relaxed self. The mother of four, she lost her second son to leukemia several years ago. She is a home-maker, a church elder, and an active participant in her local church and presbytery as well as several community service organizations. As soon as the wedding was over, Gail went into high gear on one of her biggest jobs each year, chairing and coordinating the annual CROP walk for hunger in her entire metropolitan area.

Mary Gene married young and had three children, then in mid-life found herself divorced, forced to support herself and provide for her own retirement. She moved to San Francisco and joined a local congregation that has become like a family. She works as a secretary in a microsurgery department. A few years ago she turned her many church positions over to newer and younger people to devote time to the care of and concern for AIDS victims, but at the time we were interviewing she was again accepting responsibility for many social events at her church and was again helping with Sunday school for children.

Gloria has a Ph.D. in counseling psychology. Her profession is also her ministry—serving as an individual, marriage, and family therapist in a church-based network of Christian counseling centers. She is married and has three children, the youngest of whom just graduated from college. As she says in chapter 1, her own life this past year has been full of stress. We met for breakfast one morning before she began a busy day of counseling—and we talked so long she was almost late!

Helen met with me after dealing with an exhausting hospital-board crisis. Living in a small town where her family owns a large business, she believes that economic freedom not to work requires her to volunteer her time to work for the good of others. "Not to do so would be ingratitude to God." She serves on several local and national Christian ministries and is a partner in two businesses: a small gift shop begun to help restore a declining downtown area, and a partnership that buys, restores, and sells old houses. "I ask myself, Will this make a real difference in somebody's life? If it will, then I agree to do it." Divorced for many years, she raised her son to mid-teens before she remarried, just a few months before our interview. Now her son is about to get his driver's permit. "Talk about stress?" she says.

Martha was a serendipity interview. When I spoke with Gail, she said, "You really need to talk with Martha. She does more than anybody I know!" Although Martha had a busy schedule, she spent over an hour talking with me. That's when I first heard her slogan: Shoot when the ducks are flying. "This is the most important thing I have to do right now," she assured me. Martha was formerly a missionary to Korea for twenty-five years, where she worked as a journalist, teacher, and writer. Now back in the United States, her husband pastors a local church, and Martha directs a Christian resource center. Of her four children, one is in college, one is living at home indefinitely, and one is living at home until her upcoming wedding. The fourth is married and lives in another state. In case all that's not enough, Martha and her husband also serve as foster parents for teenagers—two in the past two years.

Maxine has spent her life going around the world, one piece at a time. In addition, she works as a medical technologist, going to work very early so she will have time for the committees she also serves on. Her interests range from world missions to community theatre; she sits on the board of a bank and the county school board. Soon after our interview, she started making costumes for a community theatre production. She has been married for thirty-seven years and has raised three sons, who are all out of college. "But they keep coming back," Maxine responded. She doesn't seem to mind!

Nancy was widowed three months before our interview, after thirty years of marriage. Trained as a journalist, she had stayed home with her children until college bills loomed, then had gone back to work on a newspaper staff. These days she is heading up a consulting firm to train business and government organizations how to think and communicate effectively. The business was her husband's; when he realized illness would force him to cancel several commitments, he suggested that she take his place. He said, "If I can teach them to do it, I certainly ought to be able to teach you to teach it!" She has been managing the business ever since. Nancy deals with her grief by making new friends, cherishing old ones, and staying very active in her local church.

Shirley was married to a navy man, so she got used to raising her four children alone. She wasn't prepared, however, for divorce when the youngest was five.

That entailed moving back to her parents' town and, for the first time, finding a job outside her home. She went to work for her father's company; eventually she moved a piece of the business home where she could work near the children. Later she bought out that part of the company and started her own successful company. What made the difference for her was her own new Christian faith and eventually the faith of each of her children. "God got us through," she declares. Now her stress is that the business is growing faster than she and her employees can handle, at a time when she yearns for more free time to be with her growing family.

Notes

CHAPTER THREE:
Heavy Spirits Are Hard to Carry

1. Frederick Buechner, *Wishful Thinking* (New York: Harper & Row, 1973), 2.
2. This is a paraphrase from Mark Twain. What he actually said was "Always do right. It will gratify some people and astonish the rest."
3. Catherine Marshall, *Something More* (New York: McGraw-Hill, 1974), 38.
4. Ibid. See all of chapter 3 for a fuller treatment of forgiveness.
5. For a good discussion of two-way forgiveness, see David Augsburger, *Caring Enough to Forgive/Caring Enough to Not Forgive* (Scottdale, Pa.: Herald, 1981).
6. Buechner, 29.
7. M. Scott Peck, *People of the Lie* (New York: Simon and Schuster, 1983).

8. Ken Wilson, *How to Repair the Wrong You've Done* (Ann Arbor, Mich.: Servant, 1982).

9. Oswald Chambers, *My Utmost for His Highest* (New York: Dodd, Mead, 1979), September 15 and July 1.

10. John Baillie, *A Diary of Private Prayer* (London: Oxford University Press, 1965), 119.

CHAPTER FOUR:
One Slingshot and Five Smooth Stones

1. Amy Carmichael, *Rose from Brier* (Fort Washington, Pa.: Christian Literature Crusade, 1973), 10.

2. Adults raised in dysfunctional or abusive families can write for an excellent catalog of resources: *Tools for Recovery*, 1201 Knoxville Street, San Diego, CA 92110-3718.

3. Elizabeth Goudge, *The Scent of Water* (Greenwich, Ct.: Crest, 1965), 72.

4. See *The Way of a Pilgrim*, trans. by Helen Bascovcin (New York: Doubleday, 1979). Written by an unknown nineteenth-century Russian peasant, this book suggests one way to pray without ceasing.

CHAPTER FIVE:
I Do It All for You, Dear!

1. Kimberlee Ann Burdick, "Little Red Wagon," unpublished. Used by permission of the author.

2. Many good, humorous books give tips to make

cleaning faster and easier. Our family enjoyed *Speed Cleaning* by Jeff Campbell and The Clean Team of San Francisco (New York: Dell, 1987).

CHAPTER SIX:
Picture a Perfect You

1. Dag Hammerskjöld, *Markings*, trans. Lief Sjöberg and W. H. Auden (New York: Alfred A. Knopf, 1966), 17.
2. C. S. Lewis, *Letters to An American Lady*, ed. Clyde S. Kilby (Grand Rapids: Eerdmans, 1967), 51.
3. Richard N. Bolles, *What Color Is Your Parachute* (Berkeley, Calif.: Ten Speed Printing, 1990) is an excellent tool you can use at home to begin to discover life directions based on interests and abilities.

CHAPTER SEVEN:
Planning the BIG Picture

1. Richard and Linda Eyre, *Lifebalance* (New York: Ballantine, 1987), 16.

CHAPTER TEN:
Getting a Handle on Today

1. Gordon MacDonald, *Ordering Your Private World* (Nashville: Nelson, 1985), chap. 7.

2. Ibid., 8.
3. Alan Lakein, *How to Get Control of Your Time and Your Life* (New York: New American Library, 1990). See especially chapters 9 and 10 for a fuller treatment of this subject.
4. Ibid., 71.

CHAPTER ELEVEN:
Tips to Make Life Easier

1. See Shirley Dobson and Gloria Gaither, *Let's Make a Memory* (Waco, Tex.: Word, 1983) for many ideas to make family celebrations memory-making events.
2. For additional cleaning tips, see Jeff Campbell and the Clean Team of San Francisco, *Speed Cleaning* (New York: Dell, 1987).
3. See Doris J. Longacre, *Living More with Less* (Scottdale, Pa.: Herald, 1980).

CHAPTER TWELVE:
Watch Out for Sabotage!

1. Michael LeBoeuf, "Managing Time Means Managing Yourself," *The Management of Time: The Art and Science of Business Management* , ed. A. Dale Timpe (New York: Facts on File Publications, 1987), 31—32.
2. Don Aslett, *Clutter's Last Stand* (Cincinnati: Writer's Digest Books, 1984).
3. Basil the Great of Caesarea, c. 365.

4. Abraham Joshua Heschel,*The Wisdom of Heschel*, selected by Ruth Marcus Goodhill (New York: Farrar, Straus and Giroux, 1975), 3.

CHAPTER THIRTEEN:
A Word About Money

1. Larry Burkett and Ron Blue have written extensively about personal finances and offer workbooks to help Christians look at a total financial picture. See also Ken Wilson,*Your Money and Your Life* (Ann Arbor, Mich.: Servant, 1983); Howard Dayton, *Your Money—Frustration or Freedom* (Wheaton, Ill.: Tyndale, 1979); and Gary D. Moore, *A Thoughtful Christian's Guide to Investing* (Grand Rapids: Zondervan, 1990).
2. Jim Fain, "U.S. Is Splitting into the Very Rich and the Rest of Us," *St. Petersburg Times*, 11 September 1990.
3. Marilyn Geewax, "Living Above Our Means," *Alternatives* 15, no. 4 (Winter 1989): 7—9.
4. Lisa W. Foderaro, "Ex-executives with Nowhere to Go," *St. Petersburg Times*, 24 September 1990, formerly appeared in the *New York Times*.

CHAPTER FOURTEEN:
Coping in a Less-Than-Perfect World

1. This motto hangs over Bonnie's sink and was embroidered by her sister Deborah. Every time I

see it, I think how "imperfect" most of God's creation is—trees are lopsided, mountains are irregular. Creation reminds us that the only true perfection is to be found in its Creator!

2. C.S. Lewis, *Surprised by Joy* (New York: Harcourt, Brace and World, 1955), 213—14.
3. Gordon E. Jackson and Phyllisee Foust Jackson, *Pathways to Faith* (Nashville: Abingdon, 1989), chapters 5 and 6.
4. Oswald Chambers, *My Utmost for His Highest* (New York: Dodd, Mead & Company, 1979), August 28.
5. Ibid., September 1.

PATRICIA H. SPRINKLE is a freelance writer and hunger activist. She has served as a director of Christian education, public relations director, editor, and hunger educator, and has published three murder mysteries. Sprinkle lives in Alabama with her pastor husband and their two young sons.